TOASTERS
DON'T ROAST
CHICKENS

'In the middle of a biting cold night one January I found myself in a medical emergency clinic, in my pyjamas. Again. With a baby under one arm wanting feeding and a three-year-old hanging off the other needing help to breathe, I had to explain to an on-duty locum that our son, Ben, was a bit more than tired. He had only slept through eight nights ever, he had asthma, eczema and allergic rhinitis. He lived on a daily diet of steroids, anti-histamines, painkillers, decongestants, and antibiotics. He was profoundly deaf in one ear and hearing impaired in the other. He had related learning difficulties and I had difficulty seeing the funny side.'

More than losing a night's sleep to a fever, or a week to croup, it was losing her mind that made this school-run mum decide it wasn't good enough. Her child deserved better and she wanted her sense of humour back.

Fourteen days after she found a remedy for her son his doctor said: 'This child is well, and I'm confident he will grow out of this condition this year or within a year at the most.'

An ordinary parent learns the right questions to ask on anything from allergies to vaccinations, discovers there are only four simple rules, and one truth. If drugs worked all the time they would have done so by now, it is the way they are used that makes the difference.

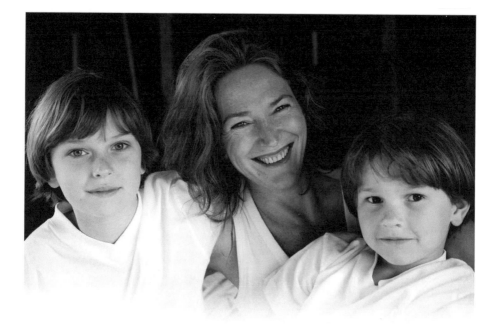

TOASTERS DON'T ROAST CHICKENS

The story of an ordinary mum who challenged conventional medical thinking and transformed the health of her chronically-ill child...

MELANIE GOW

SPRING HILL

Published by Spring Hill
Spring Hill House, Spring Hill Road
Begbroke, Oxford OX5 1RX
Tel: (01865) 375794. Fax: (01865) 379162
email: info@howtobooks.co.uk
www.howtobooks.co.uk

British Library Cataloguing in Publication Data
A catalogue record for this book is available from the British Library

ISBN: 978-1-905862-17-7

Cover design by Baseline Arts Ltd, Oxford
Cover photograph by Emma Freeman
Produced by Deer Park Productions, Tavistock
Typeset by PDQ Typesetting, Newcastle-under-Lyme
Printed and bound by Cromwell Press Ltd, Trowbridge, Wiltshire

Every care has been taken to ensure the accuracy of the contents of this book, however it must not be treated as a substitute for recognised medical advice. Always consult with a medical practitioner. Neither the author nor the publisher can be held responsible for any loss or claim arising from the use or misuse of the suggestions made, or failure to take medical advice.

Contents

'Practical guides to medicine are badly needed.' Lyall Watson, author of *Supernature*.

'Your son must be a remarkable child and you must be pleased about his healing abilities. I am delighted to hear stories like yours.' Suzi Smith, co author of *Beliefs, Pathways to Health and Wellbeing*.

'Melanie's persistence and energy in tracking down the solutions she needed for her son Ben's difficulties should be an inspiration to all parents. ...I'd like to thank Melanie for writing her book and adding, in her way, to the fuller science of healing and healthcare. I'm sure it will liberate a lot of confused, troubled, mums and dads.' Prof. Keith Scott-Mumby MD, MB, best selling author of *The Allergy Handbook*. Dubbed 'The Allergy Detective.'

'Mel's story is one of trials, hope and understanding. She heard and answered a call, one we all hear when our children are suffering ... and became a modern day heroine for us all. ...her story inspires us to be our own advocates, understanding our own illnesses, their gifts and the many possible solutions.' Matthew Carratu D.O.M.G.Os.C Registered Osteopath, Director of the Nuffield Dyspraxia Programme.

'Melanie Gow knows something that we all need to know. She has learnt that it is possible to combine alternative therapies and traditional medicine and to come up trumps. She teaches us how to dance between the two different forces for healing and to choose what is right for us and for our children. If we do what she suggests our families will be stronger, healthier and happier and we will be able to take responsibility for our health.' Julie Lynn-Evans, BA, BAC, UKCP, TV child psychotherapist and author of *What About The Children*.

'As a healthcare professional with over 15 years' experience in paediatric nursing care, I can only say that this extraordinary woman has used intelligence, motherly love and great determination to aid her child against all odds and conventional medicine. An interesting, factual read which will give mothers the courage to question the medical profession.' Avril Cartwright, SEN, RGN.

'I would heartily recommend this book to many of my clients as it reveals what I try to teach, from someone who has learnt, someone like them. Good for you Melanie.' Homeopath and NCT facilitator, Anna Foxell.

Foreword
by Prof Keith Scott-Mumby MD, MB
Best selling author of the *Allergy Handbook*
Dubbed 'The Allergy Detective'

Medical doctors seem to have an in-built resistance towards intelligent, educated patients or concerned, questioning parents of young, sick children. Somehow it seems to threaten them. Yet I have always felt that it is a major aspect of a doctor's role, to teach and inform, as well as merely treat. Indeed, the word doctor actually means teacher, not 'healer'.

It is especially satisfying to me when someone I have helped to understand key health concepts has then taken it and run with it, in the way Melanie has. **Her persistence and energy in tracking down the solutions she needed for her son Ben's difficulties should be an inspiration to all parents.** Moreover, it should show doctors that patients want to be – need to be – involved and committed to problem solving.

As Melanie points out, having just one range of simplistic and poorly understood tools (drugs) is no more practising scientific medicine than trying to cook every family meal with just a toaster. Doctors must learn to think much more broadly about health issues than is customary. Thinking 'outside the box' should not be looked upon as a symptom of flakiness or unstable radicalism, especially not when the box is so very narrow and confining. Rather it is a sign of willingness to explore, to discover, to embrace the new. New ways are refreshing and new ways may see deeper into the darkness.

For instance, it has long been an axiom of mine, that the disease is not the problem: disease is a result of the problem. Disease is Nature's way of announcing in unequivocal terms that some basic precept of health is being violated. If that violation is correctly identified then Nature herself will work the cure. Drugs are rarely required and, almost by definition, give only palliative support, not a cure. In fact, doctors are so used to this they are rather cautious of the word 'cure'.

Such a pity, since so many conditions are eminently treatable, if tackled the right way. Masking the symptoms with drugs will not help, but effective changes in the external environment, which includes diet, has shown time and time again to clear up an otherwise complex and distressing condition. What's great about this approach to health – and possibly why doctors feel so threatened –is that anybody can do it. It does not take years of dissecting corpses and memorising complicated chemical formulas to make effective lifestyle changes and benefit from the immediate improvements.

It means more power to patients and their families and I say 'Yes' to that. I have never understood why my colleagues would want it any other way. A patient kept in ignorance is forced to be dependent on the physician and I say that's not healthy. I'd like to thank Melanie for writing her book and adding, in her way, to the fuller science of healing and healthcare. I'm sure it will liberate a lot of confused, troubled, mums and dads.

Prof. Keith Scott-Mumby MD, MB

Preface
by Dr Mosaraf Ali

I really feel this book has an important message for all
parents and Melanie's journey to help her own child with his
debilitating health problems will, I hope, inspire other
parents to take responsibility for their children's health.

In my experience 80 per cent of everyday illnesses do not
need the attention of a doctor. Health is governed by natural
laws and to restore it you have to simply rectify the faults
and create a suitable environment for the body's natural
ability to heal itself.

By taking into full account the uniqueness of each individual,
physically and mentally, the context of their environment
and providing appropriate treatment, this is achieved.

Over twenty years ago I created the name Integrated Health
to express my philosophy of gathering the best of all the
traditional and conventional techniques.

Conventional medicine has outstanding advantages for acute
specific illnesses, while traditional and complementary
medicine often outshine when dealing with chronic ailments
and conditions caused by a complex combination of factors.

Melanie's story is a confirmation, in a long line of success
stories, that an integrated approach can not only treat, but

also prevent, illness and above all restore health. The body has its own intelligence and behaves like a system governed by laws of nature. As Hippocrates said 'the body heals itself, you just have to lay down the conditions'.

I personally encourage each of us to take more accountability for our own health, as a natural part of our lives.

Dr Mosaraf Ali
Director of The Integrated Medical Centre
Author of *The Integrated Health Bible*, *Dr Ali's Nutrition Bible*, *Weight Loss Plan*, *Women's Health Bible*, *Ultimate Back Book* and *Therapeutic Yoga*.

'A wise man ought to realise that health is his most valuable possession and learn now to treat his illnesses by his own judgment.'

Attributed to Hippocrates

We Ought To Be Introduced

In Africa they have a saying:

> *When two elephants fight it is the grass that gets
> trampled.*

*

I started writing this on a wonky spiral pad, in one of those
soulless rooms that smell of well-thumbed magazines and
where the chairs don't quite face each other, under strip
lights that are on all day.

I spent endless hours sitting in waiting rooms in
surgeries, A&Es and medical drop-in centres, with a baby
wanting feeding under one arm, and a three-year-old needing
help to breathe hanging off the other. My sad, anxious, little
three-year-old boy in my lap, concentrating so hard on every
breath. Waiting to be processed.

Like so many parents, I had been sure there was
something wrong with our child. More than just another
cold, at least. But everywhere I turned I was told I was
wrong, or just worrying. Or worse, I was an OAP (over
anxious parent).

That is, until we spent two days in four different waiting
rooms. First, we were told there was nothing wrong; then
there was something wrong; and finally Ben was treated. But
then, I was told there was nothing more that could be done
to make him well.

And I was expected to accept that.

Ben was three years old, exhausted, pale, thin and
depressed. He was predicted to live with severe allergies,

eczema, asthma, intermittent ear surgery and on steroids, with all their side-effects, for at least a decade, or more.

Having glue ear made him profoundly deaf in one ear and hearing impaired in the other. This makes it very hard to get to grips with phonics at school and resulted in associated learning difficulties.

All that conventional drugs could offer Ben was 'management'. For all the syrups and suppressants all the doctors, specialists and paediatricians threw down him, they could only suppress the worst effects, ease his symptoms and manage the condition.

But that's all.

They couldn't cure it, or make him better.

One cold January, I found myself in my pyjamas, at midnight, facing yet another stranger wielding the solution of an emergency prescription for antibiotics. I looked at my scared little boy; he was tired of the routine, resigned to the process, and his lungs didn't work. I decided that night that he deserved more than this, and that I wanted my sense of humour back.

I searched everywhere and in the end it was as simple as opening a book, a book with a different perspective. It took just one moment to change his fate, a fortnight to release him from the numbing drudge of living with a chronic condition, and less than a year to really put him back on his feet.

I am not here to tell you that one treatment or another is the best thing since stay-on lipsticks that actually don't leave red crescents on the rim of your mochachino cup. There was no magic bullet with Ben. What made the difference was that, as a mum, I was the right person in the right place to make integrated health decisions that were right for my child.

That cold January night, I took a deep breath and a long look at my son as an individual. I had felt all along that things were being missed. I knew his personality, what his home life was actually like and how he responded to his world 24/7. I was closest to him and the facts; I was there while his history was being made, every step of the way. I was best placed to make the links and informed choices that applied to him, personally. I could also see clearly when things worked. I could see the whole picture.

*

What I know now is if you only rely on prescription drugs it is like only using a toaster to cook with, you will never eat roast chicken.

It is not about right or wrong, or having to choose between mutually exclusive opinions. It is about balancing modern medicine's strengths with the understanding that sometimes other things work too.

Our conventional medicine is embedded in a foundation of theories, with methods of testing, statistics and sound empirical experience to prove them effective and applicable. No other system is as informed about the human body. It is very good at emergency treatment and we all still need a doctor in the house.

However, if the drugs worked all of the time they would have done so by now.

Although it is claimed that there is no certainty that alternative treatments work – in truth, there is no such promise with orthodox treatments either. Despite orthodox medicine's search for a common procedure for all people with a certain condition, any success with any individual is down to chance and cannot be relied upon.

Neither is it about monotone chanting and closing the toilet seat to improve your finances. I don't wear sandals (well, I guess I would if I could have Blahnik on them), but I certainly don't knit my own yoghurt, shrouded in crystal-fringed Kaftans waving a dream-catcher.

What I found was that the answer is not with the allopath (conventional doctor) and nor is it with the homeopath, or osteopath, or naturopath. They are all options; genuine, effective, valuable ones when used appropriately. They are all paths you can choose to take towards an integrated approach to wellbeing.

It is about making our own health our job, one that takes into account our individual uniqueness. An integrated approach looks at our environment, our behaviour, capabilities, beliefs and values, recognising the innate resources we have available to stay effortlessly on an even keel.

I found the answer is in the quality of the questions you ask. I realised it is essential to take responsibility; not in a passive, positive-thinking way, but about our ability to respond. I learnt that the Latin meaning of the word doctor is 'teacher'. And I learnt that, outside the seven minutes on average that we see our doctors for, we mums are the ones who often have to make the decisions. And some of those decisions may be ones that make the difference.

I discovered how critical it is to be guided by observation, to see what is going on and not just to look at the circumstances. All symptoms are connected. Symptoms are the rabbit produced from the hat in the magic show our immune system puts on: to focus on the rabbit is to ignore the magician.

I now appreciate that the definition of wellbeing is being well balanced and it's the immune system's job to maintain this equilibrium. Like a tightrope walker, balance is about handling imbalance. There are two categories of illness:

disease and dysfunction. We either have a bug or some part of us is not working well – life is bugging us. To divide problems into these two categories helps to decide a suitable treatment for them.

The good news is, it turns out there is only one alternative treatment to our conventional methods. Usually we treat allopathically (contrary to suffering), ie stopping symptoms by using ANTIhistamines, ANTIbiotics, ANTIdepressants, and so on.

The alternative is the 'law of similars' – to treat with the body. Neither should be dismissed, and more often our body is distressed in both ways, and a combination of the two is required.

Most importantly, it brought me to understand three overriding principles that are traceable back to Hippocrates. The first is to 'treat the person not the disease', and who knows our own children better than us? We are the people who know best the people our children are. The second is that 'prevention is better than cure' and we mums are at the heart of that role daily, especially when prevention includes good sanitation, nutrition and chilling out. The third is to 'do least harm'. I have found it more useful to turn that around and ask what I could do that would 'do most good'. Either way, as mums we naturally have in our hearts the best interests of our children.

This does not by any means make us perfect parents, but we are experts in our own children and all we need is a little information. We are smart, competent and capable, we are the generation that lives in the eye of the information age, and we have the technology at our fingertips, literally, on a QWERTY keyboard. Unlike doctors, we don't need to keep track of every disease. We can easily learn just as much, if not more than a GP, about the relatively few we have to deal with.

We have the chance to ask questions and, more importantly, find answers that mean something to us. Our great, great, great, grandmothers didn't; they had to bind wounds with toasted cheese and suck on small frogs to draw the poison from a sore throat.

I was born in Africa, a continent not just far away in airmiles but a world away in economic, educational and welfare opportunities. I respect the chance we have here in the UK to determine for ourselves our course of action. We have choices.

I have spent six years researching why what I did worked, trawling the Internet, reading the papers and attending the lectures, researching where we fit into our environment and what our actions, abilities and beliefs mean for our health. Travelling around the Third World, where I was born, to here, through applied sociology to psychoneuroimmunology, from 500 BC through medieval Christianity to conventional, modern medical practice.

It can seem like one huge mass of inconsistent information, facts, figures, opinions, arguments and counter-arguments, all backed by their own trials, tests and statistics. However, I believed there had to be a simple way through the confusion for us parents, and all this could be reduced to just a few fundamental rules, some useful tools and a short list of essential questions to ask. I wanted it never to be difficult ever again for any mother to be heard, to believe in herself and to do the best for her own children.

Busy mums like us have a lot on our plates, but healthy children eat and sleep well and they have the energy to get through a full day. They concentrate better and focus easily. They are able to enjoy those social diaries that we taxi them around. They can grow to their full potential, become self-assured, rounded humans and enjoy better prospects as they fulfil their aspirations.

What more could we want for our children? And having healthy children means life is not as exhausting for us. In fact it's fun and it is sooo worth it. After all, who do you want looking after you in old age? Someone who can lift you onto a bidet? Or a hobbling inventory of drugs who needs more help getting out of a chair than you do?

I am a regular parent with far too much housework, kids' homework, working from home and working-out by doing the school run. All I really wanted was to get it together enough to enjoy a glass of wine instead of reaching for it in desperation. I am now conscious about health, I hold it as a value and prioritise it. I no longer take my body for granted. But I am no different from you, not so you would notice down the frozen pizza aisle in the supermarket.

As parents, we agonise over the right schools for our children, read suitable books and buy well-fitted shoes, so why not put as much thought into choosing better health for them?

From one parent to another, if I can do this, you can too. I am the one who only has left-over Christmas paper when there's a birthday present to wrap and has to buy greeting cards in bulk. The unfolded laundry never makes it to the kids' drawers, and breakfast is usually still on the table at lunchtime. I am no alpha-mum, and yet I managed this. There aren't rules, there are principles and useful tools and effective questions – the questions you ask are the key to everything – that will help you to keep your medicine cabinet half empty and your glass half full. Our families deserve that.

*

1. Much Ado About Ben

One late spring day I was walking into town with our three-and-a-bit-year-old son. He ran the half-mile into the town centre, played all day, stopping only for a juice, and then ran home. He had a smile on his face the size of a melon slice.

I cried.

I cried for about three days with relief and disbelief.

This was the first time we had been able to have fun in nearly two years. That was more than half his life. For too long I had rocked Ben through a fog of night sweats and shapeless days, surviving on half cups of tea. This was the first time he had been able to be an ordinary child in so long I didn't remember ever doing it. I felt like we had our child back. He acted like he had a second chance.

Yet there's nothing unique about his story. No strange disease or tragedy to make this dramatic. Like thousands of parents, we had a child who suffered from allergic rhinitis (hayfever to you and me). He suffered from asthma, sinusitis and all the glue ear, recurrent infections and snotty, sticky, waxy things that come with the territory.

All the doctors, specialists, paediatricians, chemicals and potions known to modern medicine can only suppress the worst effects, ease symptoms and manage the condition. But that's all. They can't cure it. They couldn't make him better.

He would grow out of it, his doctor said, but added, 'It could take longer than you think, anything from seven to thirteen years'.

What he had is very common. He's one of thousands of children and adults who suffer year after year and sometimes all year round. Many people are left managing the condition for all their lives.

Ben was an extreme case.

What is fantastic and extraordinary about Ben's story, and worth telling, is his recovery.

It all began, as we remember it, with a thick cold that went to Ben's chest and turned into an asthma attack.

He was a few months old.

That first winter he caught a few colds. They all went to his chest and he stopped breathing each time. He never recovered from anything before he went down with the next one. He had chronic sinusitis. He had so many minor ear infections he thought pain was normal. He coughed, overheated, cried, sweated and looked like a pale, sunken-eyed version of a real child.

We soon learned all about the fast-lane trip to casualty, the wait for a triage nurse to send us through to a curtained cubicle, to wait for a doctor on a double shift to sign the paperwork for the ward and the houseman to sign the prescription card for the nurse to administer the drugs to help him breathe. With the nebuliser on tap, it was a long night spaced out on steroids, so high he couldn't sleep, and an exhausting week would follow as he recovered.

Somewhere around January we realised we were in a cycle and there seemed no way to break it. We had to ride it.

He would grow out of it.

Is what they said.

This story is familiar to thousands of parents across the country sitting in waiting rooms. Parents with grey faces and children with black circles under their eyes, waiting, vacantly, week after week, stuck because they can't breathe.

The descent into despair happened by degrees; it was like trying to remember what summer is like in the middle of February. You can't really recall the details of life before, you just become acclimatised. Even those friends and family who saw him regularly had to compare him to the little boy he had been a long time ago to realise how far away from well he had become. We did remember a bright, active toddler with a very inquisitive mind and a whole day full of energy.

But it was a dim memory and you are never sure if the memory is ever as real as you think.

'Kids catch colds, it's perfectly normal to have ten to twelve a year,' is the first platitude you remember. The one that makes you doubt yourself and disregard any nagging feelings. 'Really? This is just a normal cold? Well, you should know, you're the doctor, and this is my first child, so I don't really know what's normal. But you see sick children all the time, so I'm sure you're right.'

On that first trip to the hospital, a doctor mentioned Ben wasn't asthmatic. But he went off duty, and Ben was diagnosed anyway as being asthmatic.

The conventional approach to treating asthma revolves around getting to grips with equipment. It's accepted by everyone, including us, that what we essentially needed was to learn how to use an inhaler and spacer. They rushed us through the squeeze-and-breathe-in-to-a-count-of-twenty technique, and we listened hard to the 'repeat as necessary' instructions.

We swiftly mastered the art of inserting a steroid inhaler into one end of a large, plastic, double-ended bottle and placing the plastic cup on the other end over Ben's nose and mouth. That was it. Ben was a statistic, processed and discharged.

He called it his nose-bottle. It became such a familiar part of his life it was one of his first words. With rudimentary medical support we managed his condition that year. Nobody knew any answers or actually explained anything more than 'most kids suffer to some extent. They grow out of it.' But nobody said what 'it' was. We made most of it up as we went along; assuming all we had to do was whatever it was we were doing until we didn't have to do it any more.

You see the signs and try to step in quick with something that will stop it all spiralling out of control. Sometimes it worked, most times not. Ben would look like he was catching a cold, his body would react as though it was life-threatening, and we would write off another week. He would start sniffing and then show signs of a runny, slimy-green, snotty nose and within a day he would be running a temperature of 39°C and his chest would tighten. Asthma hurts, your chest and your back hurt and your stomach muscles ache from crunching with every breath. He would be unable to breathe and on a steroid inhaler repeatedly, with someone having to lie by his side every second of the next 24 hours. He became demanding, even hysterical, if you just turned away to reach for something. He was scared. He had to be sure you would notice if he stopped breathing.

We had to lie there hour after hour. We had to be looking at him all the time he was awake, and he slept fitfully.

So did we.

Every sniff made us dread what was coming. He would take the steroid and at first it would keep him going for an hour, but soon it would be only for 20 minutes. Then it became a balancing act between keeping him breathing and sending him off on a trip chasing dragons. This process would go on for three days before he would be able to eat a little dry, solid food – toast soldiers.

We didn't know when it would get better, but every time he improved we hoped it would be this time. But it didn't get better, it got worse. He was sick more than he was well. He did not recuperate each time and ended up getting worse in front of our eyes.

We had a child who cried over everything. A little Chicken Little who thought the sky was falling in when an acorn landed on his head.

Our normal lives caved under the strain and we lived around Ben's lack of health. Halfway through everything we did, even the normal supermarket run, his temperature would rise, his face would flush, his eyes would glass over and we'd have to go home. He barely made it to playschool two half-mornings a week. He coughed incessantly if he walked, and usually he had to be carried. He woke up three or four times a night, always with this uncontrollable cough, retching, drenched in sweat.

Winter colds spread into summer, too. He coughed for a whole year. By January, we spent every day managing him and his chest, trying to keep his temperature down, just getting him to breathe.

Exhausted, we lurched from heartache to anger and back again. The bright, spirited, wriggle-bottomed chatterbox who ran everywhere, spent all day playing, completed jigsaw puzzles for kids twice his age and had energy enough to drive you crazy, was gone. He was a very frightened, tired, unhappy, clingy boy. We took to a life of shifts, one of us always staying home with him.

We had been led to believe it was just a matter of coping, and we would happily put everything else aside to get him through it, if that's what was needed. Finally though, we noticed how far away from a real life we had come. How everything revolved around the issue of his chest and getting him to eat. This was no life for a little child hardly out of nappies, who should be running carefree with the wind, playing long and hard all day to be happily tired enough to sleep all night.

He had been to see so many doctors. We saw a different one every time because they were always 'emergency appointments' with the doctor-on-duty or locums, or A&E staff on shifts. Because no one knew him well, all anyone saw was a boy with a cough. And I guess he could have looked like a kid with a cold, who would get over it next week.

We heard platitudes, reiterated explanations and tired judgments to the background noise of sighing. I'm sure we were quietly filed under OAPs (over anxious parents). The very worst fate.

One doctor, who saw him soon after we brought his baby brother Harry home, even diagnosed 'sibling rivalry'.

Now we had heard every explanation – except one that made sense.

On the other side, there was a permanent clamour of people throwing well-meaning opinions and advice at us. He needs a course of iron, it's his kidneys, move countries, put him to bed earlier, have you thought of a tonic? Give him some cough mixture – as if we had not tried all this and more. We had a cupboard full of bottles of mixtures for colds, catarrh, tickly coughs, dry coughs, chesty coughs, headaches, fevers, sore throats, and all the painkiller combos.

At first, it was a little insulting. I would look at the doctor, or practice nurse, or whoever, and think: 'We have tried that and we have thought of that and we have thought that through.'

You end up frustrated and defensive and it's easier to nod your head and go away. Then you begin to believe it must be you. You begin to believe that you are tired, irritable and unable to function like everyone else because you are inadequate and not a good enough parent. You are not up to the job.

I had no confidence, particularly in front of doctors. I couldn't find the right words to reply, to explain to the experts. I know they said it was just a cold, but how bad did it have to get before it was a condition? It wasn't right to let Ben go on like this, but I didn't have more than a gut feeling to go on, or know enough to make a case to back it up. And, more significantly, you believe it is the doctors who have the experience. You rely on it.

But, nothing got better – nothing.

One day, eventually, through the fog of exhaustion, the truth emerged to stare me in the face. This wasn't right. This wasn't normal. He wasn't growing out of anything, he wasn't having several, ordinary colds. I don't know, maybe I looked too stubborn, or tired, to move out of the damn doctor's chair unless I got some help.

Whatever it was – pity, clarity – Ben's GP then diagnosed allergic rhinitis, and referred him to the leading paediatrician in the field at the Royal Nose, Throat and Ear Hospital in London, saying 'special cases should see specialists'.

The specialist said, 'Ben's a classic case,' a reactionary child with allergies and a sensitive nose. The whole experience was a relief.

The specialist and her staff were wonderful, reassuring, sympathetic and obviously experienced.

She performed a Scratch Test, injecting 12 solutions of probable allergens under the skin to test for a reaction. He was allergic to dust and its mites, and didn't like cats much either – for now. The specialist also explained that allergy-prone children can develop allergies to anything they are over-exposed to. 'There's always the summer hayfever season to look forward to,' she said.

She put him on a twice-daily steroid nasal spray, nasal drops for sinusitis, a daily anti-histamine, and one for the night, and a decongestant three times every 24 hours. He already took paracetamol like a tonic, so he was given an aspirin solution to help him through the worst bits.

We were handed a clutch of leaflets about mattresses and hypo-allergenic covers and shown a video on hoovering, and we left with these words ringing in our ears: 'Only five per cent of patients suffer to such an extreme degree. He is unlikely to grow out of it before he is 12 to 14.'

Oddly, we felt elated, relieved, almost euphoric.

Finally we knew what 'it' was, and what to do. He had been mis-diagnosed; he wasn't asthmatic. We had been treating him way too far down the line; by the time he stopped breathing, his symptoms had backed up.

So now we would begin at the beginning and this would be the start of the end.

And hadn't the staff been wonderful.

Then it sank in: we didn't know what allergic rhinitis was, and what exactly were the various problems associated with 'perennial hayfever'? It was good to know what 'it' was, name it and be given a drug routine, but what was all this trying to achieve?

It was just hayfever and quite common, right?

Like most people in situations like this we had not known what questions to ask at the time. There was a leaflet in the nasal spray box that told you how to administer it, and we had some half-remembered tip about how to get children to do it.

It became apparent how ignorant I was.

Wiping the kitchen surfaces became impossible as photocopies and printouts quickly covered them. To the casual observer it might have looked a mess of 'do not disturb' notes but there was a system, and the Marmite smears and coffee rings became like bookmarks of where I had got to in the reading. To 'become informed' I even badgered the doctor in surgery time when I had a question.

I ran hard to catch up, to master the medication routine, to care for a chronically sick child, to learn about what he had and exactly how it affected him. It ended up as a long list of little stuff: nose, ear, throat stuff, but stuff that affects thousands of us all day and night, on a regular basis.

We had a new medication routine and our new housework regime, as emphasised at the clinic. The house was damp-dusted and vacuumed with a Hepa-filter, daily. Ben got a new mattress, a new anti-allergy latex pillow covered in mite barrier to be absolutely certain. His duvet and bedding were boil-washed every week and his superfluous soft furnishings removed. All his cuddly toys were put in the loft except for one favourite Buzz Lightyear, a hard plastic Buzz with lots of buttons.

Things were going to get better, right? Surely, the harder I scrubbed and drugged, the quicker Ben would improve.

*

There was little progress after more than a month of the 'new and improved' routine. Ben was still sick. In fact, some things were worse: he coughed more, he had effectively stopped eating, had chronic diarrhoea, his sheets were streaked with dried blood every morning as his nose bled frequently from sinusitis, and he hardly responded to life around him. And he cried. A lot. Dust and mites were killing him?

One day he cried more than usual and rubbed his ear repeatedly. There was no appointment with a doctor available but he could see the nurse. She told us he had pressure behind his drum; it happened. We should just go home and keep an eye on him.

Later, he was crying and rocking and miserable but the surgery told us to come back in the morning. By midnight, he howled the house down, but the drop-in centre said: 'There's no infection. He's probably been on a lot of antibiotics, so go back home and put him to bed; he looks like he hasn't slept.'

But Ben had never had antibiotics and had had pain in his ears almost constantly for eighteen months, so something had to be wrong for him to complain, to notice the pain more than usual. But, yes, he hadn't slept well ... in nearly two years.

A doctor finally said: 'I can see his swollen glands from five paces.'

We force-fed our child spoonfuls of bright yellow antibiotics and went to see the GP every few days for about a fortnight. The GP then pronounced our son temporarily, but long-term, profoundly deaf in one ear and hearing-impaired in the other. We were to see the GP every three weeks to monitor for retraction of the eardrum, scarring, perforation and to decide whether surgery was necessary.

He also told us Ben would have learning difficulties; if you can't hear well you are hardly going to get to grips with 'phonics'.

We seemed to have reached the end of chasing symptoms. Ben had glue ear. Here was a tangible result, a chronically ill child on steroids and medication who was to all intents and purposes deaf.

*

Everyone sucks in their breath and shakes their head when they hear the word steroids. No one wants to use them, but no one can thoroughly express what it is they don't like. It is just the word 'steroids', there is an almost superstitious fear of it. Fighting through the muddle of whether it is best to use them or whether the effects are too high a price to pay, we had to remember that Ben was in a weak physical state. It is a fact that our individual cells can be in either protection mode or growth mode but not both at the same time.

We believed with short-term use they were going to do far less damage than Ben's body was doing to itself. His condition was making his life miserable and impairing his development. We had heard that in 40 per cent of cases the body's own defence system does more damage than the disease itself. On steroids, we were assured he was going to get a chance to breathe, hear, smell and taste again. Begin to respond to the world around him, to live again.

The antibiotics cleared out the persistent infection and resistant bacteria and we still assume we would never have been able to get our child to a point where he could recover fully without modern medicine. All of the gunk they stuffed up him, poured down him and made him take over those three months almost certainly were what got him through the darkest days.

However, when he stabilised, there was nothing more the doctors could do that wasn't just keeping things at bay. They could only manage the problems, drug a three-and-a-half-year-old boy sufficiently to achieve a day-to-day relief, to get him through the seasons.

And he was still effectively deaf.

Ben didn't want to be on anti-histamines, antibiotics and steroids with the threat of intermittent and potentially ineffective surgery as a regular part of his future.

Not for the next decade. Nobody would choose that as a lifestyle.

We wanted more. We wanted him well, growing, happy.

This couldn't be it.

*

You spend so much time running around the medical system you haven't the energy to persevere with something else. At some point, early on, we had attended a recommended homeopath. Only once. It was something else to drag Ben to that got swept out of the way by the circus of clinics and white coats. I figured it was pills, and pills are pills, aren't they?

I didn't get it wasn't just something else; it was something different.

I was aware it wasn't lavender on the pillow, I knew it was a holistic treatment, I even knew holistic meant it treated 'the whole of you', but it was a fuzzy concept to me. My husband did buy me a big, glossy homeopathy book with pretty pictures. However, I never had the time to do more than flick through it and leave it under a pile of unread *Sunday Times*. We didn't even have a coffee table I could leave it on.

In sickness, doctors are who we turn to.

It is the way it works.

You're sick – ring the doctor.

Make it to the appointment.

Take the prescription to the pharmacist. They're on the high street. They even open special hours and have late nights. It's all structured to work, to serve the purpose and the practice. The infrastructure that makes the surgery world go round, folds in on itself, fuelling its own momentum so fast it leaves no time for anybody to find the time for anything else.

One day I was curled up surrounded by all the leaflets, papers and relevant articles on allergy management I had gathered, scanning them.

Again.

All those soulless mocking pages I was begging to yield an answer to me gave me nothing more than more of the same information.

I could see that homeopathy book practically had a chalk outline around it from where I sat.

Right there within reach.

That book was at least something else to read.

I was sure the book would smell of fresh wheatgrass and opening it would let out the sound of whales' wombs. Pictures of test tubes filled with sincerity would decorate explanations written by people sitting cross-legged under shrines for bearded gurus in all-white sartorial radiance. But I had no other option lying around so I either read it, re-read the other stuff or watched re-runs of *Friends* on telly.

Daunted by the prospect of a whole new terminology, I skipped the introduction, the lecture on vital forces and energy patterns, the short history, the principles and philosophy and the bit on how the remedies were made. I went straight to the solution.

I looked up glue ear. I had never read anything like this.

The book described people suffering glue ear, not just in terms of the various symptoms they might have, but in terms of the stages of progression. How other seemingly unrelated symptoms were all linked, how a person felt, their likes and dislikes, how they slept and what relieved their symptoms or caused them to get worse. It was a revelation.

Each group of variations indicated a different remedy. Different ones for the different ways people responded to the same ailment. I knew people responded differently to the same sickness, but I had always supposed that was just because everybody was different.

But that's the point.

Everybody is different.

The book also explained you had to work with your body to fight the problem and you did this by using a remedy that induced symptoms similar to yours: 'The law of similars'.

I had heard the homeopath say something about the 'law of similars' that one time we went to her, but I obviously didn't listen, or I would have asked, 'How is that different to what we do now?'

I still didn't connect how the 'simile principle' differs from how conventional medicine gets things done, to how we had been doing things. Frankly, I didn't want to work that hard.

I wanted to be told what to take, how often . . .

and get a lie-in past 5.30 am.

Ben's swollen glands, night sweats, nose bleeds, the times he coughed in his sleep, his temperament, what made his symptoms worse, were all there under a particular remedy.

It was the first time I had come across such an eclectic assembly of aches and pains being linked together as if they made sense.

I figured what we were doing wasn't the huge success we had banked on and there was very little to lose.

Sometimes you just have to take a punt.

It was a low risk one and practical too; the book said it was safe, non-invasive, and non-addictive. It claimed it worked particularly with those things a doctor could only manage, or couldn't or wouldn't treat. It also said there were no side effects. We live in a litigious society and the book was written by a qualified doctor with a reputation to protect, published by a highly respectable firm, with a team of lawyers keeping them out of trouble.

Ooo maybe I shouldn't ... But what if, umm, I don't know ...

Oh for goodness sake ... it was at the very least another option.

We always need something from the bathroom cupboard in the middle of the night. Readily available without prescription in any chemist, there are directions on the click-pack and it's as easy as that to start. You don't go to a doctor for aspirin and you don't need to see a homeopath for a remedy like aconite.

I went shopping in the morning.

*

A fortnight later Ben went to his doctor for one of his regular appointments since being diagnosed deaf and our GP checked him over.

And then checked him again.

Then he got out all his new-technology toys to check Ben over really thoroughly. He put his various instruments on the desk, leaned back and paused, before he said: 'I don't know what you have done, but this child is well.'

We went to London, but this time the trip didn't seem so long and the parking was not so hard to find. This time the waiting room walls were quite brightly painted and they didn't seem to be crushing in on us. And there were crayons and puzzles on little tables and cartoons on a telly.

The paediatrician said: 'This child is well, and I am confident he will grow out of this condition this year or within a year at the latest.'

Months, not years.

When the doctor said Ben was well, he meant his glue ear condition had cleared up and he was not deaf or even hearing impaired any more. Ben still had allergic rhinitis and his histamine system still over-reacted, he was still on some of his conventional treatments – but not daily. He was well on a road to full recovery, his nose no longer bled, he slept through the night and his ribs stopped showing.

In 14 days, we'd gone from a 24/7 round of treatments and a life entirely revolving around a sick little boy, to having a well child who could face food, at least a little, and sleep at night.

It was a couple of weeks later that Ben and I were walking into town that sunny day. The day he ran, jumped, skipped, past the end of the road, down the side of the flats, over the zebra crossing and round the corner all the way into town.

He began to play with his friends, he got through a day at reception school without collapsing, and he could accept party invitations believing he would be able to go. Colour, which had long since drained away began to return to his face, and he began to smile.

*

*I am telling you them so you can make a decision for yourself,
working on the theory that all things work
some of the time.*

- It is effective. It is at its best with imbalances of physical function such as allergies, asthma, eczema and hayfever and moods. It works with the energetic system of the body and encourages the immune system's efficiency.

- It is free of side-effects. Because it works on the energetic level, it is like a radio. If the signal does not match the frequency of the body, the message passes right on by.

- It is non-addictive. Although you may end up preferring not to take any other form of medication.

- It is easy to take, especially for children. Nurturing a positive attitude to medicines promote a positive attitude to health and taking personal responsibility for it.

- It is there in the middle of the night. Because it is available this side of a pharmacy counter, you can have it in the cupboard, as convenient as a bottle of cough mixture.

- It treats the individual not the disease. Diagnosis is based on how an individual presents symptoms, teaching you to be guided by observation to make appropriate decisions.

- It treats the whole person. Physical, mental and energetic.

2. Nobody Asks a Fly to Spin Webs

Valerie Hudson, an American professor of politics and a mother, with no medical or scientific training, developed a radical new treatment for cystic fibrosis (CF) from trawling the Internet for information. After both her children were diagnosed with CF she read one report of a CF patient with cancer who had recovered when chemotherapy happened to increase a natural antioxidant called glutathione. Then she discovered in another report that the cause of CF affects the production of glutathione. She put two and two together and found that supplements of glutathione ease the symptoms of CF dramatically, and details of a clinical trial have since been published in the scientific journal *Free Radical Biology and Medicine*.

*

As parents, we agonise over the right schools for our children, read suitable books and buy well-fitted shoes, so why aren't we putting more thought into choosing better health for them?

Because that's what we go to the doctor for.

Isn't it?

But what do we do when doctors and their medicine, for any number of reasons, can't cure our ills, can't do more than manage, or even can't help?

I am a school-run mum from a mid-terrace house in middle England. There is nothing out of the ordinary about our home; we have two children, a pet, too many toys, and piles of laundry all over the house, just like most families.

Medicine wasn't – isn't – my field, but my children are. If it involves them then, just as the head of their school, or the shoe fitter in the shop, so our doctor is a resource to pull in when needed. But it should be less like a lifeline than a thread of silk in a spider's web, with the family at the centre.

I spent 35 years thinking one way, accepting a paradigm, a commonly-held belief. Nothing I have accepted as true would lead me to believe otherwise. Brought up in Africa, I lived in a country that buys wholesale into the dogma of western medicine. As a gross generalisation, everybody does. The very concept of a World Health Organisation lends weight to the idea of a western medical liberation of the global peoples from the plagues of the natural world.

We all think that way it because everybody thinks that way.

I used to be the first person who would assume, 'I need to see a doctor', and stop thinking from there on in. Run off and tell him my troubles, take the magic bit of paper away, swallow the pills and repeat as necessary.

I was one of those first-time mums who figure having children isn't going to change anything. Certainly being pregnant is just a small matter of not being able to fit into your wardrobe for a while and rethinking sexual positions. I made no concessions, ignored the demands on a body of growing another human being under your ribcage and nearly had a miscarriage. Instead of taking the hint, I rationalised that it was just one of those things and all over now ... phew. I motored on, trying to fit as much into a day as possible and wondering why I was tired, weepy and unable to achieve anything. Again I rationalised. I wasn't recovering from this miscarriage threat as well as I thought I should, and soon I was back in the doctor's surgery. I didn't stop and think; I was convinced the answer was in his hands. He would give me a magic potion and I would wake up the next morning and everything would be better again, for sure – after all, pregnancy is a 'condition'.

I sat in his consulting room and asked him to: 'Do something to put me back on my feet.'

He asked me what I wanted from him and I sighed: 'Oh I don't know, give me some vitamin pills or something.'

Which is exactly what he did.

On prescription.

I don't remember if they made a blind bit of difference or not, but that is not the point. Why didn't I understand that my body was screaming at me to slow down and it was as simple as that? Why didn't I do something sensible to help myself, like put my feet up with a magazine and a hot cup of tea? And what was I doing going to the doctor for vitamins?

Wearing leg warmers along with everyone else, I felt the pain for the gain in aerobics classes throughout the Eighties and the low-impact video Nineties. But keep fit is about the extent of what I expected to do for my own health, along with eating five portions of fruit or veg a day of course.

We're meant to leave real health to the doctors, who know so much more about such things. In fact we are considered by society at large to be irresponsible if we don't. The only thinking I expected to do was to think of going to see a doctor – after all, they do a minimum seven years of med-school so I don't have to do the thinking, right?

They are the qualified ones, with walls of certificates and respectable letters after their names. A profession is one of the highly regarded attainments in life. The profession of doctor is one of the most greatly respected. (There are children in fireworks factories and sweat-shops around the globe working, for three cents an hour, who would love a shot at it.)

General practitioners have the education, the qualifications and the habitual respect of the general public. And as a society and a civilisation we have put certain practices in place – evidence-based health policies, bioethicists, peer reviews and so on. All of which encourage our tendency not to think for ourselves.

No matter how adult or accomplished I felt I obediently handed over responsibility without a second thought and expected a doctor to be a solution. I also inevitably believed the answer he gave me was the right one, and in exchange for that veneration, the very least I expected was to be sent home with something that would make everything better – and now. I was satisfied if I walked away with a prescription; what a result.

Paediatric and general surgeon, Bernie Siegel, author of bestseller *Love, Medicine and Miracles*, says that 60 to 70 per cent of patients 'act the way they think the doctor wants them to act, hoping the doctor will do all the work and the medicine won't taste bad.'

*

Any doctor almost certainly wanted to become one for noble reasons. I know my GP reads the medical journals regularly and may even attend one or two seminars a year. When I've taken our kids to story-morning in the library, I've seen him pawing over huge books and scribbling notes to himself.

But there is no history, philosophy, sociology or cognitive and evolutionary psychology in their general training. No broad perspective or context or tools of communication. Combined with that, most of the time my doctor has to rely on his reference books, a search on the Internet, or the drug companies' brochures, PR and interpretation of statistics.

On average, the doctor has between three and seven minutes to listen, do an assessment, diagnose and prescribe. As Eric Cassell, a professor of physiology at Cornell University points out, a doctor is not trying to find out what is wrong with you, he is trying to find a symptom picture that matches a known disease. Also, his assessment of you will be based not only on medical factors but his experience of those medical factors and his negative beliefs, fears and prejudices on things like your age, sex, cultural origin, marital status and his (personal) opinion of your quality of life. This may be very different from how you see yourself. Have you any idea of the demographic picture your doctor holds about you? I can only imagine what my profile is since I got referred to see a psychiatrist once after going in with a sore throat. Diagnosis is only his perception and means the doctor's treatment could be a little off the mark.

What choice does he have? A British Medical Association poll found 92 per cent of GPs think too much is asked of them. Thousands of GPs are now refusing to take on new patients. Many point to the massively increased bureaucracy, paperwork and form-filling they are now required to do, as well as the continual organisation changes.

They spend a great deal of their time data-collecting to fulfil their three-inch-thick contracts with the Healthcare Commission. They need to process so many cholesterol checks and file as many successful take-ups of cholesterol-busting drugs and so on, till their quotas and targets and reports are satisfactorily concluded. Tick.

Boy is he busy – answering to his trust, paying the mortgage on the medical centre, managing funds and paying for practice nurses out of his own salary, because the trust will not budget for them. He is involved in schemes providing emergency care on every third day, and supervising beds in a community hospital on the second and forth weekend of every month. He is involved in academic work, occupational health or, occasionally, as a forensic medical examiner. He is trying to keep up to date, fit in training courses and submit papers, in between the inevitable inter-doctor politics, the money-conscious practice manager, the secretary and the receptionists.

The job description never stated that they should be eager to run a small business, have attended a couple of years of management training and one in accountancy, statistics, conditional probability formats, litigation and patient rights.

Then he has to deal with us, the patients.

A medical careers guide published by the Oxford University Press, *So You Want To Be A Brain Surgeon* by Chris Ward and Simon Eccles, puts it like this: 'The GP must be tolerant of people and their quirks, enjoy variety, and understand that most patients are not seriously ill but that any one of them could be.'

A doctor spends all day seeing people at their lowest, all day every day wading through hundreds and hundreds of complaints. We all offload onto him and expect him to treat us as though we are the first person he has seen that day, week or even month. There's no module for psychiatry unless you specialise and that is not what a General Practitioner is, by definition. He can never be an expert in anything and has to be an unqualified nutritionist, midwife, med-researcher and everybody's sweet maiden aunt.

Five days a week, from nine to five, every seven minutes on average, somebody dumps all their ills on him. Not to mention house calls, locum work, night shifts and the odd weekend on call. He spends his working life as a germ traffic-warden, and a third of our GPs have been physically assaulted by one of us.

To a man with a hammer all things are nails.

After all that, he goes home to his real life, where his kids are playing up, his teenagers are doing a different class of drug, his pre-schoolers are not sleeping through the night, his babies are teething. His second wife is over-worked, undergoing fertility treatment and has an expensive shoe habit to compensate. Meanwhile he is trying to fit in a social life, the neighbourhood watch meeting once a month, a visit to his aged parents at the weekends, a game of tennis once or twice a week and taking the dog for his twice daily walk. So he is not getting any sleep, his sex life is scheduled, his kids don't know who he is, and he has a drinking habit. Which he's developed because he's trying to give up smoking.

No different to most of us, but very few of us carry out government-funded faith healing or deal with people all day long who place total trust in us, and expect us to make not only them but their lives better.

Lost in a world of my own, I was jolted back to real life by a hoarse and unrelenting hack. I felt the wet spray of the globules as they caught the tip of my left ear. I came to, and realised I was in the surgery waiting room. I looked at my watch and realised we had been waiting 35 minutes for a 9.20 am appointment. I looked around. Sick people are not a pretty sight; a room full of them is depressing. They cough and wheeze into hankies, the back of children's hands are smeary and little old ladies smell of powder and perspiration; the air has always passed through too many lungs.

I thought about how long the doctor's day was going to be. What if our GP was feeling down, not in the mood or simply distracted. Doctors only have time to see us as walking ailments and often simply fob us off with whatever will make us go away happy and, with luck, well. You can also end up running from doctor to specialist to another specialist like a spider trying to pull flies out of the air.

Ben's name was called. We followed the doctor back to his room ... and we left two minutes later with the prescription.

It dawned on me, in the end we get the doctors we deserve.

If you can see how demanding it is for him, then it is pretty obvious the smart thing to do is think for yourself. 'Not thinking' may be the socially accepted norm, but it is not ideal.

If we go to the doctor without a second thought, if we believe he is the answer and if we are satisfied when we walk away with the prescription, in the end we will get the doctors we deserve. If you understand the doctor's position and its demands and the restrictions these put on his proficiency, you are obliged to recognise it is unacceptable not to think for yourself.

I hold my hands up to be counted as making every mistake in this book. I have apologised for my existence, I have adopted a submissive posture, I have gratefully accepted the prescription without question and more, oh so much more. That's why I can now say with such confidence what doesn't work.

Question: how many patients does it take to change a light bulb? Answer: what's change?

No matter how well negotiated your salary hikes or how high your company car was graded, it is not much more than hype wrapped up in well-plucked eyebrows and un-scuffed heels if you don't pull your resources in and make them work for your family. Its now about more than how boardroom-red your nail varnish is, you need to work out what you are doing there and come up with a couple of constructive questions.

Our grandmothers and mothers didn't chain themselves to railings, burn their bras and learn to sign their own cheques for us to ask someone to tell us what to do.

It is reasonable to feel a need to believe in a doctor, because asking someone for help makes us feel vulnerable. It is, however, not helpful if the doctor does all our thinking for us. If we let that happen then they do all that thinking into a tape recorder, on a referral letter, to a five-minute conference between his colleagues. Removed from us, the patient, to a discussion between employees on their programme and schedule, their department plan.

Yes, he is both busy and bored, or just badly in need of a shot of coffee, but you need his care. It is not about knowing how bad it is for him and trying not to be another demand. What was I afraid of? That I would make him angry and he wouldn't make us better?

Remember, every time someone fails to get well it is a powerful reminder that the doctor is not the one in control.

We can go to a doctor: for a diagnosis, a course of treatment, advice, reassurance, an argument, to make a point. Remember this is a world where the doctor has to assess your place in the statistics, the cost/benefit ratio, his budget and his opinion of your demographic. It could be we are the ones who have to argue for a particular test, prescription or treatment. If you know what is possible and you want a particular option it could be you have to give the doctor reason to believe you are a suitable candidate. Or, at least, make him work at reassuring you why he does not.

Imagine what you would do if the doctor sends you away without answers. Responsibility is not about taking the blame, or passive acceptance, it is about active thought within the context of your environment. It is the ability to respond. Our health, and that of our families, is our responsibility; after all, we are the ones who have to live with it.

Becoming a mother is often the first time in our adult lives when we are 'sooo' not sure of ourselves. The anxiety is exponentially increased when you don't trust yourself to make 'The Right' decision because you are responsible for another life suddenly. I pour endless hours into worrying if I feed them the wrong cereal in the morning they won't get to university – and it will be my fault.

However, we are not stupid, we are smart, capable and accountable, we too are educated, we are exceptional people – all we are missing is a little information.

It's just like laundry, you know your clothes, what suits you, how they fit, what goes together and so on. When they are dirty you put them in the washing machine. You may not know everything about how the machine works, but when you first got it you read the instructions and learnt how to make it work for your needs.

We are in the right person in the right position to know what is right for our families, and we owe it to our families.

When you put your clothes in the washing machine, the machine doesn't know more about your clothes than you do.

For all the credentials and experience offered, the truth is a doctor is not always there. Apart from those miserly average seven minutes, three days from now, he is not around and it will be down to you. You are on your own and you are the one who is faced with decisions. Some of those may be ones that make the difference, as I found out.

3. Think for Yourself

Problems are not the problem; coping is the problem

Virginia Satir, psychotherapist

*

When Ben reacted unfavourably to his DPT vaccinations it was second nature to try to be ignored than face the ducking stool and oppose the accepted practice. I am usually the first person I find hanging around to pin any blame on. It is much easier.

Insecurity sends out a scent like fear, which attracts vigorous disdain and, as I have never responded well to bullying, I blamed myself in several ways.

With reason, the immunisation programme is deeply embedded in the social consciousness as vital for our survival. It is considered the necessary and only real defence against what are seen as the predatory lions of disease constantly circling the herd of mankind, waiting to pick off the weak and infirm.

The fact that our child had reacted adversely was cause for denial more than anything else and I remember thinking 'make note to self: must do better'.

When Ben was diagnosed with allergic rhinitis that was practically a mantra. I realise there are times when the medical system is all there is to turn to and the responsible action is to get the help it offers. But, it is true it doesn't always work and there are other options you may want to integrate. The point is: it is our decision and sometimes we are the only ones who can make a truly informed choice.

*

We were referred to an eminent local paediatrician, who ran a specialist clinic for the entire county, and this was his bag: kids and allergies.

We were informed 'the point' was to sift through Ben's various symptoms to treat them one at a time, and it would give us a local specialist to manage us more efficiently.

He asked me what was wrong and when I told him what I knew he became irritated. 'You just tell me what's wrong. I'll diagnose the boy,' he said.

Confused, I thought: 'But I'm telling you what's wrong, and chronic sinusitis is what two specialists have told me he has. What do I do? Go back to square one before I knew all this and pretend I'm not the person who knows my son best? Do I just obediently recite my experience, and let you do the stuff which makes you important?'

I didn't want a simplistic, paternalistic relationship of reassurance and prescription with the doctors. But I got it anyway.

When something feels like it is not working for you it is probably because it isn't.

I could feel the pressure threatening to rise from a faint hint of hyperventilation to full-blown sulk. I knew the 'jargon' and understood the diagnosis; it wasn't just a sophisticated recounting of the circumstances. I know it is important to do as you are told, but only if you are six.

Here I was, a mere mother living with a real victim, while the paediatrician was the county expert, the private practice operator, the man in charge. He was the important person in this situation.

Not Ben, or me, or the family.

The paediatrician rode on with his agenda: 'Bring the new baby in and we'll get him started on the same thing.'

Harry was five months old and he'd been to the hospital in an ambulance a couple of times already for 'upper-respiratory problems'. He was a big baby, 11lbs at birth, and we were told it was 'normal' for a 'winter-baby' to have mucus on his chest. When the health visitor asked us the usual 'Did we have any concerns?' Well, yes, we did; his chest. Harry was 'chesty' and couldn't seem to shift it.

She replied: 'There's no dust in the womb.'

It was funny – but on the surface this seemed to make a lot of sense. We had been told chest problems would be considered hereditary in our family. They always ask if there is 'a history', and when you say 'Daddy has asthma', they nod and hmm with a 'See!'. The interesting thing is it is treated as if the two are unavoidable, inevitable and more significant, unchangeable. So it was agreed: Harry was reacting to exposure to dust for the first time and would have asthma and probably need steroids. They said big-babies always have heavy chests, big babies take time to get used to the world. It was because he was a big baby, and a winter-baby. Oh, and a boy, as 'Boys always suffer with chests.'

The paediatrician was his usual brusque self and while he put on his gloves and got all stethoscoped up, my job was to take Harry's nappy off.

He listened and weighed and prodded Harry for a couple of minutes. Then he filled out a prescription for my baby's daily steroid inhaler and said we'd find we had to use it every morning throughout the winter, starting around August, until he grew out of this. 'But best to get him started on this as soon as possible, and you'll be able to avoid the situation you found yourself in with the other boy.'

(That's Ben, our son, he has a name.)

I was dismissed. I dressed Harry, strapped him into his stroller and wheeled him home. His room is a calm hideaway, with a skylight. It's airy and restful, a haven from the world.

We had done the rounds of the services with him: emergency, general and specialist, and here we were all alone.

Settled in his nursery rocking chair, I pieced the spacer together, a ritual I was altogether too familiar with. I loaded up the steroid. I took my little baby into my arms and stared down into his clear, smooth face with the little dimples he still has when he smiles. So peaceful was his water birth, he was born without a mark on his face and his eyes closed. It took him a week to open both of them at the same time.

I looked at his face, into his trusting eyes filled with a softness which comes with not knowing betrayal. I brought the inhaler down over his mouth and held it firm while I squeezed off a couple of rounds of steroid spray. He began to struggle immediately, but I held him tight. He screamed, and I repeated over and over in my head what the clinic told me: 'It's better if they cry, because it gets the steroids into their lungs properly.' I counted the obligatory 20, I repeated as necessary, and I watched my baby panic because he could not escape. I told myself, he was frightened, but at least he was taking in the treatment and he'd be able to stop wheezing. Wasn't that the point?

I waited for it to take effect. Nothing.

Twenty minutes. Nothing.

I tried again. The whole screaming, struggling, shooting-up process.

Nothing.

It is possible that a 'preventative' steroid is not able to alleviate an existing condition, but it was what I had been given for Harry – to be used as soon as possible.

Then I remembered our GP saying babies don't have the right keyhole for steroids to unlock their problems, which could apply to all steroids, preventative or not.

I realised that no matter how well I understood the instructions or knew the point of the treatment or how well someone had explained the reason for it, I was the one in the position to judge if it worked. I was there and not the doctor; therefore it was up to me.

The noise in my head from all the directives and diagnosis and techniques and data just stopped.

I was doing everything I had been told, I was almost a control freak about carrying it all out. I had the advice of a GP, a specialist, a paediatrician and a health visitor; I didn't miss a thing. But none of them were there, right there at that moment. I had to decide what was working and what was not; there was only me when it counted.

The eighteenth century philosopher Immanuel Kant wrote an essay in which he says that an inability to use your own understanding without another's guidance is self-imposed. He points out that not thinking for yourself: 'Lies not in lack of understanding but in indecision and lack of courage.'

The doctor is the expert and so it is at least justifiable to rely on him for some things, but who are you going to turn when there is no one there but you?

I didn't have to do what the one doctor ordered, and if their prescriptive advice did not appear to work, it was reasonable to seek the infamous second opinion.

At the appointment with the specialist in London, I asked if she felt a five-month-old baby should be on a daily preventative steroid.

This specialist was adamant that a wait-and-see approach was a much better policy for such a small person, and steroids were neither effective nor appropriate.

Question: how many experts does it take to change a light bulb?

Answer: depends which expert you ask.

*

I was left sitting in our kitchen feeling a right banana, a fully paid-up member of the fruit bowl. Here we are at the dawn of the bright new millennium, two hundred years down the road of modern medicine, revelling in the longest period of world prosperity, thriving in a technological nirvana, and we rarely take advantage of this liberation to think for ourselves.

We get by day to day by paying the barest attention to the endless stream of sensory input. We depend on our subconscious memory as a survival tool to simplify everything we experience, to make it easier to get through the day. What this means is that we end up living in a world of shadows where routine creates an illusion of certainty.

When we turn to a professional, we want to buy into their certainty, as though they have a better handle on it. We are used to, and depend on, a culture of wonder drugs and miracle surgery; where the policy is to fit the individual into a ready-made profile of treatment. I felt like a fool to my own stupid desire to believe in something that was certain I would trust in it without question.

A whole team of great minds out of Harvard Medical School, led by Doctor Harold Bursztajn, wrote a book, *Medical Choices, Medical Chances,* which makes it clear that tests and treatments are inconclusive and usually have side effects, and treatment with any certainty is usually out of reach. Gerd Gigerenzer, director of the Centre for Adaptive Behaviour and Cognition (ABC) at the Max Planck Institute in

Berlin, is one of many who say we have allowed ourselves to believe in the 'illusion of certainty – such as treatments only have benefits but not any harm; that there is one and only one best treatment; that a diagnostic test is absolutely certain'. This, he says, 'is a mental obstacle toward making up one's own mind.'[1]

*

I was the second generation to be born in Kenya, a unique country in colonial history, because it was founded and handed back within the lifetime of one generation. I have tiny, brittle, black and white photographs of my paternal grandparents in full English dress, layered shirts and corsets and britches topped with pith helmets, standing outside their first mud hut. They were young pioneers on the tail end of the founding wave and chucked out as pensioners.

They left a country where there are doctors' clinics on every corner, selling panaceas from other worlds at prices that are out of this world. Private clinics, charity-run clinics, travelling clinics, clinics built with donations from bleeding hearts, and clinics set up by nurses who work nights at the government hospital. They steal supplies to sell for their own profit during the day.

The place rattles with pills.

When I was a child, the mothers of my African friends told me their elders didn't fear the Spanish with their Inquisition or the French with their guns as much as they feared the English with their Bibles and their Gladstone black-bags. You cannot torture or shoot a culture into oblivion, but you can erase it by changing it from within, by spreading hope. Buoyed by a profound belief in their own empire-building superiority and with great confidence in the virtue of their solutions, the English colonisers applied both potent preaching and pills to all people, regardless of their cultures.

The seduction of the grail of the certain chemical-control of suffering is powerful. Banking on the promise of a better world in the hereafter, I watched in Africa, as people waited in line at a clinic for handed-out answers, by people who push them convinced of their value. That was a pretty close reflection of how our family had complacently accepted what was prescribed to us by those we had positioned in authority over us and who, in turn, were led to believe they deserved that place.

In a silent, passive way, how can any of us be sure we have not become the accepting sufferers at the end of a queue of decisions taken 'in our best interests', by people who have a different agenda from our own? Like Africans in a state of grateful prayer, taking pills handed out by people who are more familiar with the statistics of the product than their patient's characteristics.

We invest financially, politically and emotionally in our medical system and our doctors. So certain are we of the tools in place to regulate what makes up the system that we feel we no longer have to decide for ourselves. We 'manage' any decision by delegating the responsibility to anyone who says it is his or her job.

Historically, the doctor–patient relationship has been based on a one-way trust and the time-honoured belief in the advantage of patient compliance. When we go to the doctor we can happily agree to being parented, because we all want our mums when we're ill. Parental reassurance has worked in medicine for so (very) many years – around 3,000 – so the idea of patient autonomy feels relatively new. Indeed it was only in the 1960s that this type of bioethics was introduced to modern medical decision-making. Drawn from philosophy and theology, it laid out the relevance of such principles as autonomy, self-determination, beneficence, and justice for the patient.

Only recently, a *British Medical Journal* editorial called for doctors to 'hand back power to the patients, encourage self-care and autonomy . . . promote the de-professionalisation of primary care'.[2]

But it's not new, Aulus Cornelius Celsus (ca. 25 BC–45 AD) was the Roman author of what is believed to be the first systematic treatise on medicine. It is the most important historical source for present-day knowledge of Alexandrian and Roman medicine. He wrote a great deal about deciding for yourself nearly 2,000 years ago, concluding that: 'What is necessary to the mind, so it is no less hurtful to the body'.

Throughout antiquity, doctors wrote treatises for the public, who in turn discussed medical problems with their doctors. The 'Father of Medicine', Hippocrates, wrote for 'the layman' at great length as long ago as the fifth century BC. It was not advice on self-treatment or even first aid; he stressed he did not want to dispose of a doctor but integrate the patient in a mutually beneficial discussion. As he says, 'The physician is the servant of the art, and the patient must combat the disease.'

We have access to water, sanitation, education, opportunity and widespread, accessible healthcare, a level of freedom never enjoyed by any other generation before us. The currency of our freedom is responsibility; we should be careful whom we give it away to. We delude ourselves if we think we are free and we have choices if, in reality, without thinking we take what is given to us over-the-counter by GPs allocated to us based on an accident of postcodes. Informed consent is not a matter of formality or a mechanism for protecting the practitioner from malpractice. In a world where the only certainty is uncertainty, where experts differ and there are consequences, we are the ones who must make the choice for ourselves. We can easily get to grips with what exactly we are dealing with and as a result we may make better choices.

*

To make responsible choices you need to:

◆ Weigh the risks and benefits carefully, is the potential benefit worth the risk?

◆ Ask if a drug is safe enough for you? Men and women metabolise drugs differently, as do children and the elderly. Know if you are in a higher risk group and always inform your doctor if you are taking any over-the-counter medication or supplements.

◆ Make sure you understand i) what the drug is for, ii) why you are taking it, iii) how you will know if it is working and iv) when to expect results by.

◆ Know where to go to report any adverse effects.

◆ Check to see if the drugs you are given are the correct ones, check expiry dates, act on recalls and safety warnings, read the patient information leaflet and ask the pharmacist if you have any queries. You are responsible for your health.

◆ Bear in mind you may want to look at other options.

Whatever option you choose, stay in tune with the body by monitoring it during the period of treatment and consider any changes objectively. Trust yourself and be guided by what you observe.

4. Painting by Numbers

There is an African proverb that translated means something like

'Ask one who has experience rather than an expert.'

*

The kitchen has a new, matt, black toaster, a four-slice, cool-wall, pop-up version, with chrome finishes. Which is interesting only because I asked more questions when buying that toaster than I did when accepting a prescription for our son.

I know what we needed a toaster for, what I wanted it to do, how I was going to use it. Whether it should be a two-slice or four-slice, take thick and thin, have a defrost button, cool wall, crumb tray or lift-up option. I knew which bread, from white to multigrain or malted, we prefer, and how long a slice takes to brown to our taste.

Most of all, I knew the toaster would only toast.

We ask questions and we spend time reading labels in supermarkets. We've taken control of our shopping.

So why not medication?

When Ben was first put on his conventional regime, I noticed, for all the doctors threw down him, Ben was not getting better. I did everything I had been told. I understood and I didn't miss a thing.

Except I had not realised we were the ones with the experience.

I was the one who was living with Ben and Harry, who knew what was going on in their lives, what their environment was like, their personalities and characters and

46

moods. I knew their past, their capabilities, their hopes, beliefs and their real and unfounded fears.

I had the experiences that put things in a context.

I had a choice: to trust others because they had the knowledge, or wise up because I understood our sons.

If we examine the environment of the medical system we are then able to be more constructive in our thinking. Learn all you can and then make sense of it for yourself. It is a more productive way to make decisions than a simplistic self-help idea of recognition and positive thinking, acceptance without understanding. The experts agree that any effective treatment only works because it treats a person in a way that matters to them. Most of the time you will be treated by a physician who is taught to be a straightforward mechanic. As Bernie Siegel says, 'In medical school we learn all about disease, but we learn nothing about what the disease *means* to the person who has it.'

In their book *Trust Me, (I'm a Doctor): A Consumer's Guide to How The System Works*, Dr Phil Hammond and Michael Mosley point out: 'Doctors cannot keep track of every disease whereas you, as the patient, with relatively few diseases, can easily learn as much if not more than your doctor.'[3]

So I piled the books up and began to read.

There were atlases of the body, with chapters on the ear, nose, throat and chest. I pored over gross pictures of growths in dermatology guides and overly intimate illustrations from anatomy books. I learnt about the HPA axis – the hypothalamus, pituitary and adrenal glands – and the thyroid and primary lymphoid organs, lymph nodes, and the Mucosal Associated Lymphoid Tissue.

I read papers which seemed more like traffic reports, about the Eustachian tube, airways, congestion and pollution.

I learnt about the circulatory, respiratory, musculo-skeletal, endocrine, hormone, digestive and neuro-systems. Then I began on the immune system.

B-cells, T-cells, Cytotoxic Th helpers and Self cells. Proteins, peptides, lymphokines or cytokines IL4, 5, 6, 10 and 13. Stimulated B cells lead to IgA and IgE which make histamine and mucosal defence.

Lymphocytes and leukotrines, antigens, pathogens, antibodies or immunoglobins IgEs, Gs, Ds, As, amino acids, MHC molecules in classes I and II, macrophages and ligunds.

I read myself into a stupor about coughs, colds, hayfever, eczema, asthma and, of course, allergic rhinitis.

I read all about allergies: what are allergies? who gets allergies? The symptoms of allergies, diagnosis of allergies, how allergies are treated.

I learnt about tests: skin prick tests, patch tests, radio allergo sorbent tests and immunoelectrophoresis-serum tests.

I learnt statistics. One in three people in the UK will develop an allergy at some time. If you have one parent who suffers from allergies, the chance of you being the one in three is a further one in three. If both parents are affected, the chance is increased to two in three. Four out of ten school children have at least one allergy. One child in five has asthma. Over one million people have a food allergy. An estimated six million people have eczema. Over nine million people have hayfever.[4]

A staggering 30 million of us live with one or more of The Big Three: asthma, eczema, or allergies. One in three people in the UK suffer from a chronic (meaning long-term or frequently recurring) illness or disability.[5] One hundred and fifty thousand asthma attacks a year are severe enough to be admitted to hospital in the UK every year and more than 1,600 people die. There were 35 million prescriptions for inhalers in 1996–7, at a cost of £400 million to the NHS.[6]

After all the anatomical explanations, diagnosis methods and numbers, do you know what I started to pick up?

One word.

One word started to bother me.

Management.

They know all about the physiology, immunology and endocrinology of the whole issue, and the bottom line – the last amazing thing they can do for you – they can tell you how to manage allergic rhinitis.

After all that, we can do no better than just live with it.

As a kid, I loved to watch a comic troop of guinea fowl blustering through the tall dry grass to nowhere in particular. African folk tales always cast this plump, scurrying chicken as the most ridiculous bird and the butt of everyone's trickery. They are like polkadot balloons that burst into flurries of panic even at the sight of their own shadows. Mystified by their own actions, their reaper-black eyes blink blankly in their vivid scarlet and electric blue, bony casque heads. Like a town council meeting, they squawk indignantly all day about how 'it shouldn't be allowed'.

Knowing they were called guinea fowl did not make either them or me any smarter. They were still dinner.

Cataloguing, categorising and collating are strangely human activities; no other species keeps journals or index lists. Knowing what something is called is nowhere near to understanding it for what it is or being able to deal with it.

Information is not insight.

Analysis also creates a distance, a lack of engagement, like spitting into a glass. We swallow several hundred times a day but if you spit into a glass and examine your saliva are you then going to be able to drink it? You could find out what its chemical make-up is and be able to make an accurate, detailed, objective record of it, but this won't help you swallow it again. And yet we do all the time.

Doctors have learnt to classify rhinitis into categories: seasonal, perennial, perennial nonallergic and vasomotor rhinopathy.

They can discuss the disease processes – from the inhalation of the antigen to the discomforting signs and symptoms. Sneezing, both blocked and runny nose, itching of the nose, mouth, eyes, skin, impaired smell, sore throat, headache, loss of concentration, chronic cough, wheezing, and so on.

They can identify precipitating factors: irritants, inhalants, household allergens (dust, dust mite, feather, animal dander), outdoor allergens (pollution, mould spores or tree, grass and weed pollens).

They can summarise the natural history of allergic rhinitis and list the complications – sinusitis, orthodontic problems, otitis media (middle ear infection), the list goes on.

Doctors can describe different 'treatment modalities' (ways to treat) such as environmental controls (lots of lovely housework and special bedding), inhaled and systemic steroids, decongestants and antihistamines – with various different classes each of them.

They can talk the talk of topical applications, speak of cromolyn sodium and, in addition, tell you of its use in patients with 'concomitant' asthma. They can discuss everything from indications for immunotherapy down to allergic/non-allergic conjunctivitis at great length. They can even give you their view of the impact of allergic rhinitis on the quality of your life.

But, whatever paper or guide or advice I listened to, they all ended the same, with a system or process of managing the condition, to manage the impact on the life of our child.

There's that word again: manage.

I looked up the word.

'**Ma'nag/e** *v.t.* & i. Handle, wield control, regulate (with *can* or *be able to*) cope with' – *Oxford English Dictionary.*

But coping is not a solution, let alone a cure.

Imagine what it's like to know all that we know and it still amounts to nothing more than a management programme.

*

Then they mention, almost in passing, 'judicious use'.

'Don't over-use the medications; they become less effective the more you use them.'

'But my child needs them, you said that's what you have for him.'

'Use your judgment and don't over-use them.'

'So, the more serious an attack becomes, the more I'll have to use the treatments, and the less effective they will become. This will make the symptoms less manageable and therefore they will get worse?'

'You also have to bear in mind the comparative acceptability of the side effects over the damage the condition is doing to the child.'

'His name is Ben . . . Sorry, what's that about side effects again?'

'As with everything, nothing to worry about. Not everybody suffers all of them at any one time. There is a list in the small print at the end of the leaflet included in the packet, if you are interested . . . Oh, don't let it worry you; most reactions are mild, if they occur at all.'

Have you ever read the possible side effects just on a bottle of decongestant from a high street chemist? Feeling sleepy or unable to think clearly, dry mouth, burning, stinging, redness or itching. Headaches, runny nose, appetite stimulation, weight gain, hormonal disruption, growth retardation, not advised for patients with epilepsy – the list goes on.

And somewhere in there is something known as benign prostatic hypertrophy. Which I am fairly sure is not a prize you can put on a shelf along with your school swimming cup.

*

Progress has been swift and, at times, great. Our grandparents grew up in an age without antibiotics, open-heart surgery, organ transplantation, pacemakers, kidney dialysis, hip replacements, keyhole surgery, MRI or ultrasound scanning. The range of treatments, diagnostic techniques and methods of preventing disease that we now take for granted was simply unknown.

This is progress, but the age old question 'Do we really do this with full knowledge, wisely and judiciously?' needs asking.

There are a growing number of Multiple Drug Resistant (MDR) diseases. The miracle of antibiotics has been abused, making them less effective. Vaccines are an imperfect art and there has not yet been one successfully manufactured for a parasite – for example the malaria parasite, which kills 1.5 million people a year. Viruses don't respond to conventional medication, there is no cure for chronic degenerative diseases and most forms of allergy or auto-immune disease, and no effective management of most kinds of mental or psychosomatic illness.[7] The list grows of drugs which don't work or cause equal problems to the disease. There is a growing concern about how many conflicting medications are building up in our bodies, needing more medication to treat the effects they cause.

Do we understand what exactly it is that doctors, the system and the drugs can actually offer? Food labelling is now rampant; not just content, calories and chemicals, but how it is produced and who produces it and whether they are paid fairly or not. Shouldn't we be asking more questions about the drugs we dose ourselves with than what we wear, eat or plug into our kitchens?

In amongst all the reading I did I found one particular statistic interesting: despite there being more than 170 published clinical trials, there is no consensus on the best drug for the initial therapy for middle ear infection or acute otitis media (AOM).[8] Which is what Ben had, and thousands of our children have, all over the country, and will continue to do so. This made me realise I didn't know that much about the drugs being prescribed or why they were prescribed or what the chances were of them working.

Acute otitis media (AOM) is one of the most common reasons children end up at their GPs. Most children experience at least one ear infection by the time they are seven years old. AOM is one of the most common reasons for prescribing antibiotics. Ben had been prescribed antibiotics and we believed they had cleared out the infection. But research has proved it takes seven children with AOM to be treated with antibiotics for it to work for one kid. Six of every seven children with middle ear infection either do not need antibiotics as their first type of control or will not respond to antibiotic therapy.[9] This is the figure officially known as the NNT, or Numbers Needed to

Treat. There is no way of knowing which one it will work for, just that your child has a one in seven chance of antibiotics curing their earache. Our chances of benefiting from any treatment is often well below 50 per cent – now they don't tell you that at the surgery door.

NNTs are of course relative figures; it is not always true that a high NNT is terrible, because it depends on context. An NNT of seven in a fatal condition could be good odds – one person in seven could be saved, but it is a handy piece of information and is all too often deliberately excluded. Of 359 articles published between 1989 and 1998 in five major journals, all included a relative measure of how the drug reduces health risks, say Jim Nuovo and Joy Melnikow at the University of California, Davis. But only eight reported the more significant figure of how many people a doctor would need to treat before one of those patients sees the benefit.[10]

French physiologist Claude Bernard (1813–78) also pointed out a statistical ratio 'means literally nothing scientifically and gives us no certainty in performing the next operation'. His point is that there is no way to determine if the next person to be operated on, or treated, falls into the statistically advantaged group or not. There is no way to know if you are the one in seven, or ten, or one-hundred-and-eleven who will benefit from any procedure.

Despite a huge amount of data that proves women assimilate, process and respond to drugs differently from men, most drugs are tested on fit young men who, I am sure, pretty-up the place for the nurses who carry out the trials, but make a mockery of every trial for painkillers used in labour that have never been tested on women.

*

Every time I learnt something, got through a step or a stage, another one revealed itself, in an endless pursuit of a solution. The more I chased down the details, the more elusive it became. It becomes a game of reductionism, and in an attempt to define absolutely what it is you are dealing with, you find every account of allergies, eczema, asthma and their management excludes or omits others.

Until the result of knowing so much is not to have a more complete or accurate picture, but to see the gaps highlighted. Like painting-by-numbers with the red pot missing, at the end, when you hang it on the wall, the unpainted parts stand out.

Just knowing that the antibiotic we gave Ben only had a one in seven chance of being the right antibiotic for him, brought into relief how much we trust the drugs. You could put up with a GP having an off day, if you were sure you could get out of the system what you needed – a prescription you could have faith in. The last blanket of security is always that the drugs can be relied upon.

And yet, Lynne McTaggart, in her book *What Doctors Don't Tell You,* points out that 'after many years of wracking my brain, trawling through the information on thousands of drugs on the market, I cannot think of a single category of drug besides antibiotics that will do anything more than what drug companies call "maintenance" '.[11]. Certainly drugs developed to treat chronic diseases, such as asthma, eczema, allergies and arthritis, at best do no more than alleviate symptoms and usually prove to contribute to making many people worse off than they were before.

It seems that trying to match every patient's needs, regardless of their creed, colour, age or gender, with a limited range of inflexible solutions is an exercise in gambling. Any success is at best random and unpredictable. At its worst we should remember that gambling is not a low-risk investment. The odds are always against winning.

5. A Question of BRANDing

Cynics suggest it starts at the top with 'the biggest and most powerful drug company on the planet [whose] investments snugly coin in profits at the rate of $1 million an hour'.[12] In a world in which 'large transnational corporations have effectively surpassed the jurisdiction and authority of nation states',[13] the pharmaceutical industry is the most profitable on the planet. At the end of 2002 the global market was worth $406 billion and growing at a rate of eight per cent a year. Certainly it is an industry with 'a clear interest in medicalising life's problems'[14] and finding new problems with patentable cures.

But we do still have the ability, the free will, of veto. Any medical circumstance requires consideration. The first tool for starting your own line of enquiry when faced with a modern medical matter is an appropriate acronym.

BRAND

B – Benefits, what are the benefits to me of taking this treatment?

R – Risks, what are the risks to me of taking this treatment?

A – Alternatives, what are the alternatives, and is no treatment one?

N – NNT, Numbers Needed to Treat for the treatment in question

D – Duration, how long can I expect to be on the treatment?

A list of, and a tool for calculating NNTs are freely available on the web at www.jr2.ox.ac.uk/Bandolier

We are like addicts hooked on the holy grail of chemical certainty. We are wholly invested in our methods of treatment, convinced they have been proved conclusively right, by all the research, tests, trials and the creation and interpretation of statistics. The clinical distance designed to keep experts from emotional involvement combines with the lack of time to offer anything other than a standard package doled out to everyone, no matter what their circumstances. It would seem there is so much faith in the infallibility of the system that we are unconcerned about effectiveness, side-effects or the consequences. We are confident all these can be treated with yet another pill, convinced this is the right and proper approach.

Until, in old age, we have become a hobbling inventory of chemical consequences.

I don't know about you, but for me it is not good enough that we are given medication, long term, with serious side effects that requires judicious use, when the end result is not healing. This amounts to treatment without end and a lifetime commitment to chemical control of disease. Which is at best imperfect and, in the end, may be the cause of degenerative chronic conditions, or rack up fatalities.

Not healing.

That is asking a toaster to roast chickens.

Not to dare criticise this is to say we should favour a culture in which mindless compliance is OK and accept that when we are hardly functioning we have the best treatment.

Thinking that my children, our children, are destined to end up in the same place down the road feels cold and unacceptable. A bleak future that sounds like a relentless, dull roar inside my head that I can never get away from.

I believe we deserve better. My children certainly do.

I believe now that the ideal could be higher.

The antibiotic may have cured Ben's infection; it's considered to have a significant level of success in children with allergies. But, it is important to note, none of his other treatments had a chance of even doing that. Not one of them.

If what we do is flawed, and it is, then there must be a rule to follow, a couple of basic principles that make better use of what we have available and what we do with it. We need to go back to the basics, back to principles that are traceable all the way to Hippocrates. Yet relevant today.

*

THE 1ST RULE

Be guided by observation

6. Be Guided by Observation

One African story is about Mwanzi – they are often about Mwanzi – who found a weary fish eagle collapsed in his compound one hot morning. He lived far from the lake and had never seen a bird like this; he exclaimed 'You poor thing how were you allowed to get into this state?' He trimmed the eagle's talons and cut its beak and clipped its wings. 'Now you look more like a bird,' said Mwanzi.

*

I left Africa and closed the door on it for good. Put it behind me as no more than a happy playground I grew up in. I certainly learnt Africa was looked upon with varying degrees of liberal pity. The first time I returned to Africa was on honeymoon. My husband dared to take me 20 years into my past, back to my childhood. But I discovered it wasn't a trip down memory lane to a forgotten museum of the past, but a relevant and vibrant present that would also pass on 'The 1st Rule' to me.

Remember that cosy couch in the gloom of an English winter where I opened the homeopathy book? The cures described in those pages were made from plants, animals and minerals. Names without patents I could recognise even in Latin, like *Coffea*, *Sulphur* and *Euphrasia Officinalis*. They told of a time when ordinary people felt connected to this earth and each other; they certainly weren't names like Cromoglycate, terfenadine, astemizole or fexofenadine.

*

We were two metres underground and ten metres into an old mineshaft. It was cool and the tunnel entrance was like a full moon behind us. With all sound from outside cut off, the thick air was alive with quiet clicks. Our guide silently motioned us to crouch and crawl under a collapsed support through to the end of the tunnel. We stood up into a cold, dark void. The blackness above us began to move, the clicks grew insistent and something brushed through my hair.

We flicked on a torch.

Caught in the beam a foot above our heads were thousands of bats. Two-inch, big-eared, and very rare Mouse Bats.

Disturbed, they took flight and swarmed past us, so near their membrane-thin wings skimmed our faces on the way to the sunlight. They were almost silent and as we turned to watch, they became translucent against the sky. We were caught in a whirlwind of chiffon skin fluttering down the shaft of light to the heat of the African day.

We were about an hour's walk into the last rainforest in East Africa. Without knowing it, my understanding of the spontaneous nature of healing began there, under the flight of bats fleeing to the leafy canopy of Kakamega forest.

I couldn't help feeling I was incredibly privileged; it was exhilarating to be in the middle of so much life. Primal wisdom permeates East Africa. It is tangible; you can feel it in the air you breathe. It seeps under and around everything, relaxed, untroubled by the missionary zeal and medical aid frenzy that pervades the daily world of the people. Beyond all the Bible-bashing from orange-box podiums and authorised drug dealing, there is a profound sense of life going on with or without us humans. It is about scale, and it is large, and in it we are as significant as the ant. This perspective, in size and time, is what everyone raves about Africa but can't quite put a name to.

Deep in the heart of Africa and unable to afford materially or culturally what the west offers, the Luhya people of Kakamega forest are pretty near the end of the queue. Just past the reach of commercial interest but in front of food parcel drops and drought, they miss out. So they are not waiting for someone to tell them where their salvation lies.

Sociologist Robert Merton described this path of rebellion as one way to adapt to any blocked opportunity. Unlike other ways of responding, rebellion is a group response, looking to replace the typical goals and institutional measures of an unequal system. As the global modern medical body has become so big that it is no longer flexible enough for many, it is inevitable that some people will find it does not hold the answers it promises. Ignored, at the end of a tether and disillusioned, they turn away, unnoticed by this monster passing over them. Instead, they become resourceful, and to find productive, practical treatments within their control, for their own community.

According to functional analysis, this indicates a society failing to maintain itself. Those who no longer benefit from society stop blaming themselves and respond by taking a stand, which challenges the stability and perpetuation of that social system.

The Kakamega forest is a 2,400 square mile island of what used to be a rainforest that stretched clear across the continent of Africa. Less than 400 years ago it lay virtually unbroken from the Indian Ocean to the Atlantic. Oblivious to its greater significance, as no one has shown it has any value, it is being logged relentlessly for firewood, and to clear land to cultivate and graze livestock. With the natural resources diminishing with the available shade, itinerant men are reduced to offering guided walks to infrequent tourists.

In a place where people live on 60 pence a day and a banana costs half that, you need the patience to wait for any money to turn up.

When tourists are the occasional travelling missionary or the medical aid worker on a year's assignment, business is slow. The guides are used to sitting all day under the canopy waiting for a meal ticket, but, one long hot morning, they began to breathe in rhythm with the forest. They began to see the minutiae of wildlife that exists oblivious to the immediate needs of humans, and to sense the Earth harbouring powerful secrets that few people remember how to use.

Kakamega is one of the last natural habitats of the colobus monkey, and while they remain they are now being studied. Not by biologists or naturalists or any 'ists' with armfuls of degrees and large grants, but by a handful of locals without paper or pens. People who were just sitting there long enough to notice the details.

The Luhya are not strangely painted or postcard tribespeople, they are very like you and me, they share the same concerns about education, economy and health. Building on groundwork laid by the Kenya Indigenous Forest Conservation Project, the Kakamega Environmental Education Programme (KEEP) was set up by the forest guides, headed by a Luhya called Wilberforce Okeka. He became curious and began by tracking the monkeys in order to make the next guided walk more profitable – flushed with their first sighting, excited foreigners tip more heavily.

Soon Wilberforce became familiar with the characters of the individuals within the group and began to know their habits. He noticed what the colobus did when they got ill, and what they then ate. In the meeting place, when the guides swapped funny stories of their tours, Wilberforce noticed the guides talking about sick monkeys foraging with purpose and making themselves better. He asked the other guides to watch out for the sick colobuses and report back what they ate for a stomach-ache from eating rotten bananas and so on. They soon realised the colobus went in search of the same bark, leaf or seed for relief for their bad tummies, each and every time.

Wilberforce decided they should try it for themselves. He and another guide (under protest, he claims) ate a rotten banana to give themselves stomach ache, and then chewed or sucked the same plant chosen by the colobus, while the others looked on and giggled.

But Wilberforce Okeka 'proved' a cure.

Through following the colobus' every waking moment and sleeping under their trees at night, the local community of Kakamega learnt the secrets of the forest's pharmacy as our ancestors did thousands of years ago. In the haven of the shadowy gloom there are 300 species of birds, 45 per cent of all recorded butterflies in Kenya, seven species of primates, and other mammals, as well as snakes, reptiles and untold species of insects. Many of these animals are found nowhere else in East Africa because similar habitats no longer exist. With the help of the forest, the guides discovered for themselves the knowledge already known and tested in nature, by nature.

The Luhya don't have a sophisticated bank of diagnoses to draw on, so they have had to reinvent this process too. They look at each patient as an individual and listen to the patient's description of how they feel, assess their displayed symptoms, ask questions about how this change in health came about, and figure a possible cure to match the account. Before illnesses had names, the symptoms were observed and treated and we matched the cure to the individual in the absence of a term for the illness.

They are learning to treat their illnesses by their own judgment. I was fascinated by the raw simplicity of being guided by observation and to treat exactly, and only, what they were looking at.

They have found the solution to their own problems from within their community and themselves and they have learnt the first principle, the one we need to start with in every case. They are taking their lead from what they see and are 'guided by observation'.

They have little choice but to look at physical reactions in detail, and follow the symptoms they see in both the primates and themselves, and the responses to each remedy. The tribe diagnose without medical directories and treat without patents, and they are successful despite the absence of conventional healthcare provision. They say it works for them because they have nothing to go on but what they see.

We used to know this; similar secrets were known by every mother in the developed world, too. Our grandmothers would have been forced by lack of access to anything else to be 'guided by observation'. They would have known what they were looking at too and the resources of the herbs and vegetables in their garden and the value of a little chamomile tea for a colicky baby. What's more, they grew it themselves.

Practitioners of traditional Chinese medicine claim they can tell a person is going to be sick before the person themself knows or even feels he is sick. Personally I am usually wiser in hindsight but, when I pay attention, I can tell when my children are heading for a rough patch. Learning to really look, not just watch, has helped me to tackle things early and usually a simple regime change, a pyjama day or even a cuddle can head-off whatever it is. The Luhya had lost the knowledge of their ancestors just as we no longer know the roots of our own medical system, how we got here, and why we use fexofenadine instead of fennel. We've just forgotten what it is we are looking at and how to do it. But if they can learn to look again then surely, with our education, economic advantage, and high living standards, we can too.

*

Soaked in curdled, vomited milk and sitting in the brushed nylon seats of a small Vauxhall in 37 degrees has to be one of the more unpleasant ways to find yourself considering the truth of needing to look closely at what is going on.

Ben complained of stomach-aches and had diarrhoea, something he'd suffered from for months. Even when he was three he would come and ask for a nappy and then hide behind the sofa every time he needed to go. He point-blank refused to sit on the toilet because he did not trust his bottom wasn't going to fall out every time, and he wasn't about to have it flushed down a bowl, no way.

It's not like I hadn't tried things. I had already read, tried and shelved every suggestion you can find in toddler training books, and doctors told me it was nothing more than 'toddler tummy', 'growing pains', 'attention seeking' or simply 'imagined', or offered invasive tests for Crohn's disease. 'Anyway it's most probably because he isn't eating much' and, as he drank milk happily, we should 'top him up on that'.

We took a short holiday in Greece, where he threw up regularly, two or three times a day. Thinking it could be the change in milk I stopped giving it to him and noticed he stopped complaining of stomach-aches. His specialist had said an allergy-prone body like Ben's could develop an intolerance to anything it was over-exposed to. Maybe he didn't take too kindly to milk.

After four vomit-free days I decided to test it.

He was asking for a drink anyway, so I gave him a bottle – I was just dumb enough to do it while travelling on a remote road in the rented car miles away from a running, let alone hot, water supply.

With that unmistakable smell clinging to the air and my thin, summer top pasted to me and going cold, it became crystal clear for all to see his symptoms were linked to milk.

As the people that really know our children, we are best placed to take a good look at them, discover what is really bothering them and work with it. Within five days, Ben's stomach had cleared up completely, and within three weeks he happily hopped up on the toilet.

Luckily we never had to pursue the Crohn's test.

Simply observing exactly what was going on with Ben guided me towards the right solution for him. The Luhya had taught me to stop looking for a label that fitted, and really look. They taught me what it really means to be 'guided by observation'. What you are looking at are symptoms, but we have to get to know exactly what we are observing so we can be guided by it.

*

7. Perverted Evolution

' The reason why the universe is eternal is that it does not live for itself; it gives life to others as it transforms. '

Lao Tzu, Chinese Taoist philosopher, 600 BC

*

To much fanfare and self-congratulation the genome code, the 'Book of Life', was opened. However, behind all the noise there was a murmur of disappointment. Despite our self-proclaimed complexity, we found we have fewer genes than a humble grain of rice. Rather than the 100,000 plus we expected to find we are revealed as making do with as few as 30–45,000, about the same as a squid. But this suggests that we have a small genome as a concession to our complex immune system. If we had any more genes, our bodies would be crippled by autoimmune disease because our immune cells wouldn't be able to recognise the huge numbers of proteins genes churn out.

Scientists moaned a bit more about how our relatively small genome may hinder our ability to adapt to environmental change, and how the genome has to come up with other ways of performing new functions. Since we can't add genes, it is our immune systems that may be all that stands between us and going the way of the dinosaurs.

If there is one single thing we can judge everything by, our immune system is probably it. Any truthful understanding of health begins and ends with our immune system. It is a rich, intricate and highly developed, flexible system with a remarkable innate and resourceful intelligence for the continuance of our very being.

So it makes sense to treat symptoms, but what are these symptoms we must observe to guide our choice of treatment?

As a general rule, they are what we observe; we see them as signs of illness, to make any judgment about a course of action. We create 'a symptom picture' which we match to a diagnosis. Blah, blah.

But, seriously, what are they really?

I discovered you can buy a book on symptoms and disease patterns but that will teach you literally nothing about yourself as a human being.

A list of around 30 major different diseases from colds, through shingles, stomach ulcers, diabetes to Aids share a common range of around 30 symptoms – like fever, chills, muscle pain, fatigue, headache. The one overall thing that this collection has in common – is us; *we* are the common denominator. That one thing they all have in common is a human immune system. With some small degree of individual variation, it is our immune system's fight that produces symptoms, not the diseases themselves.

We produce symptoms, in response to a problem.

They are not produced by the problem.

Symptoms are in fact signs of a fight our immune system is putting up for us. So when we observe symptoms, what we are looking at is our immune system; we are looking at ourselves. Our immune system is an innate, sophisticated, defence organisation, without which we would be rich pickings for the invisible predators or pathogens (germs, viruses, bacteria, parasites and fungi) that always surround us. It is all we have between us and them – viruses, bacteria, larger parasites, and other 'invading' micro-organisms. Some it allows to integrate, to become a part of us for mutually beneficial reasons, but the purpose of the immune system is to maintain a boundary between self and 'other'. Identifying what is a part of who we are and what is a potential threat, an invader, an enemy; micro-organisms that are not PLU, 'parasites like us'.

It is our immune system that defines us.

Our immune system is our identity, our physical 'self'.

We have two distinct processes that do this for us: the 'basically incredible' and the 'frankly miraculous'. The first is the 'innate' – the bit that is a part of us; the second 'adaptive' – the flexible friend that is capable of learning.

The innate, or passive, defences are our physical barriers of the body, like skin and mucus. The largest organ of our body, skin, is our main barrier between us and them (pathogens both good and bad). All the sweat and sebaceous gland secretions create a surface with a Ph value that is too low for most bacteria to survive in. Think of the infections that can fester when your skin is broken; without skin, we would look like the walking wounded. While mucus can smother bacteria so they can't get a grip and slip on out, some body fluids contain a natural antimicrobial chemical all of their own, while others are dynamite, like lysozyme, literally exploding bacteria. Once trapped, neutralised or blown-up, we get rid of bugs by sneezing, coughing or crying, or through bodily fluids like spit or wee. Now you know why.

But if life gets a bit too much – you know, when demand outstrips our resources (like parenting does most of the time) – we get that thing that we all know is bad but can't quite define: stress. This *stress* alters our biochemical composition, and our Ph balance is thrown. Now you know how to respond to 'I am not stressed.' You can snap, 'I am just a little alkaline, that's all.'

Anyway, if the scales are tipped, the sneaky little micro-organisms have a chance to slip between the gaps in our system. So, in response to these rather underhand attacks, we evolved the 'frankly miraculous' immune system, known as 'active' or 'adaptive immunity'.

The security company with this contract is the white blood cells, which are produced (like all blood cells), in the bone marrow. They are smart cookies; they are able to recognise, identify and remember specific 'non-us' organisms and develop exclusive immune responses to each and every one of them, known as antibodies. Don't worry, no jokes about them being married to unclebodies, they are more like anticipators: fast, furious and carrying a double 0 licence to kill.

There are a couple of them, both sounding like science fiction special agents: lymphocytes and phagocytes.

Phagocytes, 'the cell eaters', come in two families, polymorphonuclear phagocytes, PMNs, (bet you're glad you know this) and macrophages, 'big eaters'. PMNs are like vultures, they circle the periphery and get to enjoy the more scrappy pus-forming bacteria and anaerobic and inflammatory conditions. Whereas the macrophages are like hyenas: they are particularly good at scavenging; they even consume the body's worn out cells, and they can engulf and digest foreign invaders. They squirt a wide variety of powerful chemicals, and play an essential role in activating one of the other scary characters, T-cells.

T-cells are lymphocytes. There are three in the family of T-lymphocytes: 'helpers' or 'inducers' – regulatory T-cells whose job is the wreckage of beaten up viruses; T-suppressor cells do what they say on the tin, turn the helpers off when they have done their job. Finally there are the more dramatic cytotoxic T-cells. Programmed to fight specific intruders, they are predators loaded with chemical toxins which kill micro-organisms in cells. They blow holes in intruders, allowing fluids to force their way in, causing the intruder cell to explode.

B-lymphocytes (B-cells) – belong to a group of proteins known as immunoglobulin (Ig). B-cells are specialists. Each one is programmed to make a specific antibody to fit a particular enemy. As you can imagine each B-lymphocyte is a complicated little sucker, with approximately 100,000 immunoglobulins on its surface, designed to identify specific antigens, and found in different parts of our body, from tears to intestines. They are divided into five major types: IgA, E, G, M and the last one, D, well, nobody knows what it does. Now isn't that intriguing?

OK, now you can take a deep breath.

I could tell you all about how genes produce proteins like interferon and natural killer cells but the basic summary is that we have an entire savannah-range of honed predators and scavengers. All of them working in tight symbiosis with the circle of life.

The only catch is that everything else is keen on its own survival as much as we are, and, only one of us will survive. Our immune system is all we have between us and the malevolent self-interest of other organisms with which we live on this planet. It is a constantly evolving race for continued existence. They invade, our immune system studies them, never forgets a face, and the next time it comes across them we've got the slippery little germ's number. Of course, the pathogen is in this to win too and its one-celled primitive instinct to live fuels the development of its own safeguard. Selection pressure (aka evolution) produces this cycle between the competing organisms, us and them, which is on-going and without end.

The story of antibiotics is a great demonstration of this – hopefully it will make you treat them like a proper grown up, next time.

One day we were watching Ben singing for the school harvest festival service, which is held in a garrison church in town. Painted onto the walls around the pews are epitaphs to local soldiers from both world wars. Along the top is listed how they died and, with a futile repetition, most of them died not from the fight or from wounds, but from infection. Tragically, one of the biggest, septicaemia (blood poisoning), more often took hold following successful operations on their injuries. It was infection, not the war, which ended up killing so many soldiers.

Sent to France to set up a battlefield hospital lab during the First World War, Scottish-Canadian physician Alexander Fleming (1881–1955) saw at first hand how the enemy artillery was an amateur assassin in comparison to the humble bacteria.

On his return, Fleming went in search of antibacterial agents and, as he was a sloppy worker, he had a pile of Petri dishes in the sink that had been there for days (this was pre-dishwashers). When he got around to straightening them up he spotted mould growing just off centre in one of the dishes, and all around the mould the bacteria had been killed. As early as 1500 BC, there are records describing the use of moulds and fermented materials in the treatment of diseases. By the time the United States entered the Second World War, penicillin's benefits were well known, and the government recruited more than 21 chemical companies to produce it. From January to May 1943, a comparatively small amount of only 400 million units of penicillin had been made; by the time the war ended, US companies were making 650 billion units a month.[15] Many of us are here only because penicillin saved the life of one of our parents or grandparents. Penicillin's ability to cure people of many once-fatal bacterial infections has saved so many lives that it is easy to understand why it was once called a 'miracle drug'.

However, produced by a fungus, even this natural drug has proved at best flawed – it is now known to contribute to immune system and hormone disorders, allergies, psoriasis, diabetes and even developmental problems[16] – but worse than this, it has proved mortal.

Something Fleming himself predicted.

Just four years after drug companies began mass-producing penicillin, microbes began appearing that had recombined genetically to resist it.[17]

Bacteria are the oldest living things; there are thousands of species; over 1,000 could fit across the head of a pin and some bacteria divide into two new bacteria every 20 minutes.

Penicillin kills by preventing some bacteria from forming new cell walls. One by one, the bacteria die because they cannot complete the process of division that produces two new 'daughter' bacteria from a single 'parent' bacterium. The new cell wall that needs to be made to separate the 'daughters' is never formed.

Antibiotic resistance occurs because not all bacteria of the same species are alike, just as people in our own families are not exactly alike. Eventually, the small differences among the bacteria often mean that some will be able to resist the attack of an antibiotic. They are the ones who grow to breed – three times an hour.

Usually a harmless passenger in the human body, *Staphylococcus Aureus* was the first bug to fight penicillin, and by 1952 as much as three-fifths of all Staph. infections were penicillin resistant.[18] A penicillin-resistant pneumonia surfaced in a remote village in Papua New Guinea, in 1967. At about the same time, American military personnel in Southeast Asia were catching penicillin-resistant gonorrhoea from prostitutes. The American National Centres for Disease Control and Prevention agency also reports that in 1992, 13,300 hospital patients died of bacterial infections that were resistant to antibiotic treatment. It is the natural fight for the survival of the fittest.

New antibiotics are constantly being sought, and they have been successful, but the repeated or continued use of antibiotics creates 'selection pressure'; the resistant bacteria survive, enabling the growth of antibiotic-resistant mutants.[19]

In some cases the situation has become alarming, with some pathogenic strains popping up that show multiple resistance to a broad range of antibiotics. In a report in the *New England Journal of Medicine* on 28 April 1994, researchers identified bacteria in patients that resist all available antibiotic drugs.

*

Along with believing that statistics were meaningless, French physiologist Claude Bernard was most renowned for combining 'experimental skill with theory and had a valuable talent for noting experimental results that were not in accord with existing ideas'.

An American physiologist, Walter B. Cannon (1871– 1945) got to name this theory 'homeostasis', but it was arguably Bernard's greatest contribution to rational understanding of the human race. Bernard nailed the definition of 'wellbeing' by pinning down the essential formula for survival: he worked out that our cells function best when immersed in a fairly constant concentration of chemicals, within a narrow range of temperature and osmotic pressure (the force of a dissolved substance on an impermeable membrane).

Like onions, to last a long time we have to be kept in a fairly continuously even pickle, in a lightly sealed jar and in a larder-like even temperature.

To do that, our immune system is capable of learning about other worlds, exchanging information, recycling, reclaiming and reducing exactly what is needed to maintain our perfect eco-world. Our immune system is so green it practically has a Soil Association mark on every cell.

Some scientists have gone so far as to describe the immune system as another sensory organ distributed throughout the body. It is like our five senses in that it is hard-wired by nerve connections to provide the brain with information about our external environment and internal environment. It is a system that is so sophisticated it can tell the difference between a cell from another person and the identical cell in your body (which is why transplants require immune suppressing drugs). Our immune system is in fact, perhaps more importantly, personal, they are 'us'.

Symptoms are like the rabbit in a magic show; to think the rabbit is the main act is to overlook the skill of the magician. For that reason it seems counter-intuitive to the process of 'health' to spend so much time focusing on the rabbit. The immune system is a beautiful performer who is always polishing the act and symptoms are just the thing you find yourself looking at.

*

8. Walking the Tightrope

For there to be mosquitoes there has to be swamp first.

Old African saying

*

The image of Africa is of bug-eyed, bulge-bellied famine victims on a charity poster, the recipients of 'gift certificate goats' and cast-off clothes. In return for monthly direct debits, we learn of Africans from charity letters. That is what we understand by 'African'.

With all those hours Ben and I spent sitting in waiting rooms, we had a lot of time to stare at those two-colour, A5 posters promoting flu jabs and prostate checks. It occurred to me that illness has the same PR company as Africa. The image is that health is about a bleak battle with bugs, just as Africa is all about the starving and the victims of drought, exploitation and war. However, that's like looking at the poster and thinking it's the full story.

Africans are also poets and politicians, farmers and lawyers, teachers, miners, shop keepers, IT consultants, economic migrants, entrepreneurs, taxi-drivers, doctors, rangers, vets, peace protestors, tribespeople and office workers, fathers and mothers. The sick and hungry are simply the clear problems that have obvious solutions.

Here, in the wealthy and industrialised nations of the twenty-first century, infectious and parasitic disease accounts for less than 0.5 per cent of all deaths, whereas, according to a report by the University of Exeter for the DoH, a full 50 per cent of visits to doctors are for complaints without an ascertainable biological base (there is no diagnosable reason for the malaise). That is a whole lot of people who we don't have a clear answer for.

Infectious and bug-related diseases are obvious, diagnosable problems for which we actually have solutions. But what about the gripes and grumbles that have our doctors confused?

Illness can be divided into two groups. There is the time when there is an obvious invasion from a slippery little sucker: and that is disease. Then there is the complicated: and that is known as dysfunction – some part of ourselves does not function optimally. The good news is that all illness falls under one or other of these two definitions: disease or dysfunction.

I began to understand the distinction: if you are suffering from a cold, you have a virus; if you suffer cold feet your body's system is out of whack.

Pollen is a normal part of life and plenty of people are unaffected by it, in fact it is common not to notice it. Even though an allergy to pollen is triggered by something in the environment, it is our individual immune system that makes a mistake and isn't working normally. A post-viral rash is, as it sounds, linked to an ambush by a pathogen. Eczema, although again affected by our environment, is our skin – us – reacting badly. We are ill in two distinct ways; we either have a bug or some part of us is not working well – life is bugging us.

Disease or dysfunction, that's it.

Obviously, if this categorising were simple then doctors and drugs would be much more successful. Some cases are straightforward, either one or the other. But, more often, we are a mix of both and are more challenging because we are all life-long works-in-progress.

Like the millions of African lives that cross paths, cooperate, fall in love, fall apart, laugh and sigh, dream and wake up to another day, there are that many intricate interactions going on inside our bodies. Giving us plenty of room for things to go wrong: this is the recreational ground of dysfunction.

*

You may think all this seems to have very little to do with the busy lives we all lead. So busy being busy, having a busy diary till August next year, can't stop, gotta catch-up, see-you-next-Tuesday, grin-and-bear-headaches, colds and stuffed noses. What do you mean chronic fatigue? Don't give me those fancy new names for tired. We're all tired. Yet being busy is part of the picture: we do get coughs and other crazy little things we can't see but know are there, however they are hobos and we are very capable of moving them along on a normal day.

They are 'disease', and the difference between whether they get to move into the neighbourhood or not comes down to how well we are handling our busy lives. It's a good thing if you're thriving on the rush, but when the plate spinning, juggling, time and space bending, never-being-able-to-finish-a-thought life get too much, you and I call ourselves stressed. Feeling stressed is something we all know is bad for us but can't really say what it is. Nowadays when scientists refer to this pressure we experience, called 'stress', they usually mean it is not something in the environment or something in us; it is the product of the combination of both of these on a person; in other words, stress is how any experience we have affects us.

If we are feeling just peachy then usually we are 'functioning' well and don't have a problem with your average bug. However, although stress is a vogue term so liberally used it seems to have no sense, it is very real and causes bodily changes such as an increase in the hormone cortisol, and a decrease in testosterone. Both of these have an impact on the action of insulin, which regulates blood sugar and so on. Even psychological stress has a physical, causal link to the immune system.

To our immune system any stress, whether a bug or just life bugging us, is very real. The one line summation is: it's when the demands on us outstrip our resources.

It is in the gap between demands and resources that disease and dysfunction find room to manoeuvre. Both these wraiths of infirmity have an easier time settling in, and the body has a hard time staying in shape, in this void.

One way to grasp this is to see what doesn't go on when we are well.

The presumption is that specific germs cause specific diseases. If this is true then they should cause those diseases, and only those diseases, each and every time they enter into the body.

Germs like diphtheria, pneumonia and tuberculosis are often found in perfectly healthy people who do not have, have never had and do not subsequently develop the disease.

No disease culture has ever been made with normal healthy living tissue, despite medical theory declaring that germs attack and destroy healthy tissue. Neither has a germ ever been known to multiply in normal tissue in a lab. In a series of experiments in 1921 with 62 volunteer navy personnel, researchers attempted to cause a flu infection using every possible method; injections of blood from active flu cases, spraying germs into the volunteers' throat and on their food.

The results were? No reactions.

I find that interesting.

We can be, well, disease free.

We can be healthy and carry a disease but not ever develop it.

We can also carry a disease like, say, a herpes simplex virus, and only get any trouble from it when we are a bit run down.

Over 50 scientific studies dating back to the 1920s have found a person can carry the herpes simplex virus and not be affected by it until they are under 'stress'.

We can also feel ill and have 'nothing wrong' with us.

But we can also feel run down and actually become more susceptible to catching something.

The first case that documented this phenomenon linking stress to an increase in infection was in 1919. A Japanese scientist called Ishigami published his work on tuberculosis in schoolchildren.

Using a crude immunological measure – the ability of white cells to destroy foreign bacteria – Ishigami was able to relate a decline in immune function to periods when children were experiencing high levels of 'emotional excitement'. Which was further linked to an upsurge, in this case, of tuberculosis.

He concluded the emotional stress was responsible for the decline in immunity, which, in turn, made the children vulnerable to disease.

Any disease can enter a body, get the moving van unloaded and successfully settled in if the body is a run-down area in need of regeneration. Having squatters brings the place down a bit and so its harder to get back to being a desirable neighbourhood, which again makes you more vulnerable to other squatters.

As Ben found, when we are stretched we are more vulnerable to infection, which in turn eats away our perfect functioning, so we can end up with both disease and dysfunction.

*

There is a potential for the whole thing to spiral out of control, and it often does. You know what it is like if you have had too many sleepless nights, there's no food in the fridge, the laundry is piling up and you don't remember where the Hoover is because it's so long since you had a chance to use it.

These physical demands, and psychological and emotional anxieties, all go towards to us getting ill, often by altering our susceptibility to disease.

We are familiar with the idea of viruses, bacteria, parasites and their mates, disease, but I am not convinced we are nearly as sure where the line is between them and our bodies not functioning well.

I pretty much figured that asthma, eczema and allergic rhinitis were 'diseases' and had to be treated by being stopped. But all three are a body that is malfunctioning. Yes, asthma (particularly Ben's) is triggered by an irritant, like cat dander or pollen from outside in the environment but (and this 'but' means 'take note here') normal lungs do not spasm in contact with the same substances. Nothing from his environment, 'outside' himself, was actually making Ben ill; he was doing it to himself. It is Ben's system that has learnt not to handle some things well, that is 'dys-functioning' – not that he is under attack from a foreign species.

To survive involves growth and protection, but our individual cells can be in either growth mode or protection mode – not both at the same time.

When everything is going well, our bodies are growing and maintaining themselves so well they are practically humming along. When we are under pressure, cells are forced give up growing and take on a defensive posture. This means that what resources we would normally use to grow get diverted to protecting us. In short periods of brief stress, we are designed to cope – in the flight or fight mode – but for long periods of stress, our energy is diverted from growing and maintenance. If the stress response is on continually, like stepping on a hose, the signals travelling over your body will not get the proper messages through and will not be able to function at 100 per cent.

Lingering in the 'protection mode' can in due course destroy the body's defences, not least because normal replacement of protein – the main working parts of all cells – cannot happen.

Protection is not just about defending ourselves physically against a pathogen but also about behaving protectively, emotionally and we can even function defensively. Experimental evidence shows the body goes into the same protection mode when we experience grief, feelings of failure, suppression of anger, and other 'negative' emotions. With the same consequence: an over-secretion of the immune-suppressing chemicals, like adrenalin and cortisol.

A cellular biologist, Dr Bruce Lipton, expands this further, saying: 'Even body posture can be changed to brace itself against trauma, either real or perceived.' Besides physical bracing, prolonged stress can also result in 'psychological bracing', so we even begin to form beliefs and values that we feel protect ourselves.

The field of applied psychology claims that there is an ever-greater neurological investment in our brains up six levels starting with our environment and going through our behaviour, capabilities, beliefs, identity and our role in a community.

Dysfunction can begin, and have consequences on, any or all of these levels, because pressure can come from, or be felt in varying degrees on all, or at any one, of these six levels.

It can happen in the little spaces in our cells.

Matter is an illusion, according to 1984 Nobel laureate Carlo Rubbia. What seems solid is actually the reaction of a particle in a confined space. In an atom, the electrons are bound to the nucleus by electric forces that try to keep them as close as possible. Restrained, they whirl around – orbit – at velocities of around 965 kilometres per second. They look and feel solid because of this, like a rotating fan appears to be a complete disk. All the electrons in the atoms of a cup have the same orbit, but a different orbit to the electrons of the coffee.

Every solid particle of matter is composed of more than 99.999 recurring per cent empty space. The void between two electrons is proportionately as large as the space between two galaxies.

Our bodies are proportionately as empty as intergalactic space.

Chemicals cannot think or organise themselves or other chemicals without being instructed by something. In other words, as Doctor Keith Scott-Mumby MB, ChB, author of *The Allergy Handbook*, wrote, 'There is no way that the biochemical plasma or our bodies could contain enough information to organise and control a living organism.'[20] Our total genetic material can easily fit into the bowl of a teaspoon. But, what is actually important about our genes, their intelligence, occupies no physical space at all.

*

The house is a tip; I have boys, so there is Lego everywhere. I argue with all you mums with the pink version of the species, Lego is worse; it hurts way more when you tread on it barefoot than Barbie doll shoes. Boys are smelly, dirty and messy, messy in a way that means every cushion is on the floor, the laundry bins are full and I wish wet towels were the only thing on the bathroom floor.

After a bank holiday weekend, the job of cleaning up has me reaching for Belgium chocolate coated raisins and day time TV, in a classic avoidance strategy. But the science bit says, the second law of thermodynamics governs the activities of life. This says that the natural state of matter is chaos and that all things need to run down and become random and disordered. Living systems, like us, consist of highly organised matter, which is created out of chaos. Order is maintained by bringing in energy from outside to keep that system going. Like housework, it's the energy that maintains the order.

This is an observable pattern in life, like hoovering, we need energy to make any of the chaos of our life operate. All around us are countless vibratory patterns of activity, informational fields, which we don't consciously detect. You can see this book, because you are connected to it through an electromagnetic field, in which the vibratory energy of light is travelling. Electromagnetic fields are integral to the organisation of all material systems, from atoms to galaxies. They underlie the functioning of our brains and bodies. We exist as regulated and informed energy; we need these information fields to hold us together. It is within this that we function: all our little electrons whirling around and held in fields of intelligence or information. Biological information fields are huge amounts of data many times greater than the combined total molecular complexity of our physical substances.

You don't have to understand the details to know in amongst all that there is a whole lot of room for individuals to differ considerably in perception and interaction. As within a population of a continent, there is a ton of room for individual things to go wrong and create 'dysfunction', and holes for disease to slip through.

*

What does this tell us about the way we treat ourselves? I don't mean a-warm-bath-with-candles-and-a-glass-of-wine treat ourselves, I mean medically treat ourselves. I came to recognise that treating Ben was less about fixing him and more about restringing him, like a cupped hand of loose pearls. We had to thread all the opalescent, beautiful pieces of him back together before we had a whole, unbroken circle.

Most of the time I am only just managing that law of thermodynamics and producing order one step ahead of the chaos. I can't adjust the colour and brightness on the TV let alone stay well adjusted. I am the one who makes an arrangement for Tuesday and another one for the 8th of May without realising they are both the same day. How well adjusted we are is the key to staying on an even keel; like a tightrope walker, balance is about handling imbalance.

Bear in mind that any treatment system that just focuses on the disease is only seeing half the solution. Any system that just deals with the environmental factors is missing at least five other levels, and any system that treats chemically is concentrating on one teeny-millionth of the whole.

We don't change from health to disease all at once or in bits and pieces, but organically on a scale between disease to dysfunction – and healing can take place at different levels.

*

- Illness is about as personal as it gets. It is an imbalance in our biological and neurological system. It is sometimes a simple dynamic but more often it is not related solely to one thing.

- On a scale of one to ten, if ten is perfectly healthy, it is not often that anyone rapidly slides down the scale to having a disease. Health is a state of balance. The process towards both health and illness takes place over time.

- There are two categories of ill health: dysfunction and disease. Disease is an attack from something 'outside' of ourselves. Dysfunction is about the 'inside' story of ourselves.

- Symptoms are a sign that you are trying to restore order to your internal universe, whether the struggle is with a bug or within yourself. All symptoms are part of the whole and should be read collectively. If you deal with only one of them you probably will not solve the problem.

- Virtually any symptom associated with disease can be present in dysfunction, because it is our imbalance that produces the symptoms, not the illness.

- Functional illness can be the first sign of a disease. It can represent a very early stage of disease or it can simply mean that because the person is 'stressed' they are vulnerable to infection.

- Illness is more often due to dysfunction than disease. There is more scope for dysfunction within all the occasions when demands outstrip our resources. Some dysfunction doesn't have a medical label or a diagnosis profile.

- One way to think of it is that the organs, tissues, or systems of your body don't work as well as they should, but the compromised structure remains normal. Like asthma, eczema or allergies, for example.

- Lots of symptoms that we assume are everyday stuff can be the first signs of imbalance. Like disturbed sleep patterns, stomach problems, malodorous bowel movements, lethargy or fatigue, muddled thinking, hyper- or hypo-activity, if the body runs either too hot or too cold, or if the skin takes on an unusual hue.

- The tools of modern medicine tend to be much more effective for diagnosing or treating disease than dysfunctional illness. Standard interpretation of diagnostic tests and exams often miss dysfunctional illness, a result of functional disorder resulting in a pathology.

9. That's no way to treat malady

Using an electronic device which shows which part of a brain is being used, neuroscientist Benjamin Libet's experiments in 1985 showed that when a person decides to move a finger he experiences that decision 500 milliseconds after there is neural activity in the motor areas – we start to lift a finger before we decide to. We process perhaps 14 million bits of information per second. The bandwidth of consciousness is around eighteen bits. This means we have conscious access to about a millionth of the information we use to survive.

*

I love drifting off to sleep at night to the sound of the washing machine, tumble-dryer and dishwasher whirring away; it sounds like the heart of the house unconsciously getting on with the job while the family sleeps. It seems an echo of a promise that was the fifties housewife's dream – when the automation of chores was meant to replace the labour-saving device that was, until then, known as 'wife'.

I remember being at my grandmother's and idling through perfectly preserved piles of magazines, decades of back copies for recipes from canned goods and tips to get rid of odd stains.

I was drawn to the adverts, bold statements in red splashed across the drawings of white goods, promising to unshackle women. I imagined my grandmother dreaming of nothing more to think about than getting up half an hour early to put her make-up on. Spitting into her mascara cake to soften it and coating her eyelashes in a magnifying mirror quickly before grandpa saw her without 'her face'.

When I was allowed to leaf through them, I could almost hear Bill Haley and the Comets rocking around the clock in the background. There were articles about *On The Waterfront* with Marlon Brando pulling out of the shadow of un-American activities, and pages of models in an era of siren simplicity in women's fashion. I particularly remember a striking redhead actress from Minnesota, Arlene Dahl, who started a highly successful cosmetics and lingerie company. She launched the first patented bed-cap since 1925, setting the tone for a generation of women. My grandmother loved the layers of overlapping petals of nylon net ruching because they hid the hair-setting pins that held together her newly liberated indulgence in femininity. She even took to the rubber version for the beach.

Of course I wake up to the changes in our lives as women; we live in a time when department stores no longer sell bewitching boudoir ensembles and 'the cap' has a new meaning. Magazines have moved on to selling celebrity as an escape, since chores have never been eradicated, no matter how many powerballs scrub our roasting pans and rim blocks freshen up our bowls.

On a dull day, I can suffer from dirt-rage, (mostly because I don't get out enough to feel road-rage, I think,) and unleash an immeasurable fury at the boys. I know it's true that in 100 years' time no one will know how much housework we've done, but there is still a certain amount of grease that needs an elbow for a civilised existence. And how much mess can boys leave in their wake? However, most days they are smart enough to keep me too busy to notice till bedtime, when it's too late to yell. So I end up in a comforting fog of unrelated thoughts as I clear up every day.

I remember thinking that I had lost something I believed in, I had accepted without question the certainty of treatments for what seemed like forever – I was now finding that assertion so terribly flawed, all at once, not in little bite-size, digestible bits. I had not even known I accepted the conviction of modern medicine as conclusive. Just because you believe something doesn't mean that you know it. It is not enough even for your belief to be true. Philosophers would say that in order for a true belief to count as knowledge, you must also have reason to suppose your belief is true.

Some of what we 'know' is just something we believe in. Some of what we believe in, we don't know we do. Some of what we do know we believe in, we don't have a whole lot of objective reason to believe is so.

Around seven o'clock one night, the kids were getting into their pyjamas and I was trying to find the pages in the homeopathy book that would explain what kind of treatment homeopathy was.

Instead, the book fell open at a chapter of little potted ancient histories. Distracted by demands for a bedtime story, I left it open there.

Around nine, I heated up do-for-supper soup, and sat down with the past, the pages opened in front of me. I was tired, and I figured history would be easier to get my head around than theory. I have ended up spending a great deal of time with these old guys and found that many of them reassuringly said the same things. I got very fond of them, but that night they were names on a time-line, not friends yet, and it all seemed to have begun a very long time ago. A contemporary of Socrates, circa 460 BC, a Mr Hippocrates (yes, he of the Hippocratic Oath) did some work that is the foundation of our medicine. He was the very first person recorded in our culture to separate medicine from magic and religion. He founded the very radical idea that disease was a result of natural forces and environmental influences, and not divine retribution. For that alone, he deserves his founding title, but he also believed the purpose of medicine was to help our natural healing power to cure ourselves. After closely observing nature, Hippocrates announced that there are two possible ways of curing: by the contraries and the similars. In fact, he is credited with developing The Law of Similars. The Roman medical writer, Aulus Cornelius Celsus, is famous for relying on this approach, in which the principle is to treat illness with something that produces similar symptoms to the problem.

The 'if you are tired, the remedy is sleep' principle.

The cat ever so politely rubbed up against my leg to remind me I hadn't fed her. Chores stopped the headlong charge towards the goal of completing the chapter, a mental breather. Distracted by the thought that our cat might not like what I had to give her, as it was a new flavour, so who knows, I slipped into thinking about the homeopath we'd visited. It nagged at me that she had said treating like-with-like was how homeopathy worked. It had been the only explanation she offered at the time, but I was too focused on getting the treatment into my grubby hands to do more than nod agreeably, pandering to her wish to be heard.

So why was this so important?

I settled back with the next guy who has been dead a very long time, a well travelled and ambitious Greek physician, circa AD 130–200; Claudius Galenus, or Galen of Pergamum, appointed physician to the gladiators at the age of 28.

His position gave him great opportunities to see inside a working body as he dealt with 'horrific maulings', as the texts put it, and so was acquainted with sliced-open, living, pulsing people. This gave him an edge over his contemporaries as, at that time too, vivisection was outlawed in pretty much all the known world. His diagrams of most parts of the body are so vivid you can almost picture him hovering over a freshly wounded gladiator and licking the end of his quill with relish. 'Hold Spartacus down, I need to see a little more of his iris...!'

His terminology has influenced western medicine, and is still used today. In fact, all the parts of the eye – cornea, pupil, sclera and so on – were named by him; tonsillitis, appendicitis and pneumonia, all his. Galen was prolific, cutting edge, he never wasted an opportunity to see inside a body; alive, cadavers or primates, all were fodder for him. He also devoted much of his energy to rationalising and codifying existing medical knowledge. He quickly rose in the ranks and went on to serve no less than four emperors. As a writer on medicine with a working knowledge of the anatomy, he also brought philosophy back into the debate, to help him win his many arguments.

This one man's ghostly tendrils of influence have reached through the dark ages and into our practices today. As recently as 1959, a Dr Haynes was summoned before the Royal College of Physicians in London, a body that plays a pivotal role in setting and maintaining standards in medical practice. Apart from its role in examinations, training, education and research, it also advises the government, the public and the profession on health and medical matters.

It summarily dismissed Dr Haynes for considering Galen's work fallible, and he was only readmitted after he submitted a written withdrawal of his position.[21]

Between Hippocrates and Galen, you have nearly covered the whole of our medical influences from physiology to philosophy.

Hippocrates devoted a great deal of time to exploring the idea of balance in a human body. Although he wrote extensively on the 'contrary to suffering' principle, he established it was to be used in extreme cases. Galen, too, believed in applying contrary remedies to 'force out diseases'; however, he devoted much of his work to expanding this theory and called it 'Allopathy'.

I looked up from the book, it was about eleven o'clock and I needed to put the dishwasher on. I was probably going to forget all of this by the morning, and was any of it relevant anyway? As I moved the pans and plates around to squeeze the last cup in, I ran through what I'd read to see if anything stuck in my mind.

There it was, floating in my chore-occupied brain.

THERE was the most essential piece of information.

Forget the old geezers and their dates and achievements; it is about approaches to symptoms, relevant still today.

One approach is to treat symptoms with something to produce the opposite effect in our bodies. Conventional or modern medicine is known as Allopathy, which means 'contrary to the suffering'.

It treats through suppression or control, 'applying medicines to obstruct the disease'. Using drugs to suppress symptoms; '*anti*-depressants', '*anti*-biotics', '*anti*-inflammatory', '*anti*-pyretic' etc. Or produce the opposite of symptoms, using a substance to cause constipation, like aluminium hydroxide to treat diarrhoea.

The other approach is the opposite of this: to treat symptoms with something to match the effect in our bodies. Homeopathy means 'similar to the suffering'.

'Like-for-like' remedies are intended to support your body's own defence system. The remedies used to cure are known to be capable of producing the same symptoms, or similar effects to the symptoms, in a well person. If you have a cold with streaming eyes and a runny nose, the remedy may be *allium-cepa* or red onion, known to produce a runny nose in a healthy person chopping one for the pot.

Galen never understood the circulatory system of the body. He did find that blood vessels carried blood; however, he believed blood flowed from 'creating organs' to all parts of the body, where it was consumed, and no blood returned to the heart or liver. When he cauterised a wound and it stopped bleeding, this made sense to him of the idea of contrary treatment. Treatment of a suppressing nature worked and in the context of his time would have produced better results than what they had been doing.

However, this has become a habit over the years to the point where we don't even know we are doing it and therefore don't even think to look at it any other way.

I had assumed the two ways of tackling illnesses were modern medical intervention or no intervention; fill out a prescription and get on with it, or let nature take its course. When I began this, I didn't want to know how it all worked, I just wanted our kids to get over their infections and to breathe properly. I assumed it all worked the same way as conventional medicine, but different; different in a 'dippy-hippy' way, but nevertheless intended to stop the symptoms. Alternative treatments were nothing more than variations on a theme of intervention; alternative intervention.

At no time, in all the reading I had done, had anyone compared these two opposing theories. Certainly I don't think this is obvious and it shouldn't be lost in some dull history section most of us don't read.

'Anti-suffering' is the underlying principle that informs and guides our medical system, our philosophy of treatment and our drugs.

Gimme this straight, I've got a boil wash to fit in before midnight.

- The GP treats allopathically – contrary to suffering.

This results in stopping an attack from a pathogen like a virus or bacteria, but is also used to suppress your body's own defences.

- The alternative is to treat with the symptoms – like-for-like.

This is thought to work with your body's own defence systems, and is particularly effective for imbalances within the body.

Why isn't this comparison of principles more widely known, more widely expressed? Why isn't this the first point brought up when discussing treatments? Why don't we understand this about our conventional treatment philosophy?

This is the most important distinction we will ever need to know to make a rational, informed consideration of any treatment.

Why don't we, the great-unwashed public, know this?

Does a treatment work with me or against me, and which approach do I need most for my specific ailment?

We all know if you have a cold that the mucus you produce is your body trying to expel something; it is normal and usually beneficial as it is a mechanism the body has evolved to drive out something that might otherwise spread to the rest of the body and damage vital organs.

Same with a cough; it's a defence device, a means for your body to exorcise the demon bugs. Fevers are another 'evolutionarily selected biological defence mechanism'. Although it is a good indicator of illness, it is actually a universal reaction from fishes to mammals that we generate in direct response to infection to overcome it. Like all organisms, bacteria and viruses work best at an optimum temperature, fever is designed to make it so hot the pathogens are boiled alive. Except where a fever is about to cause febrile convulsion, experiments have shown suppressing a fever can actually hinder recovery from infection.

It should be obvious to a four-year-old that handicapping the soldiers on your own team doesn't give them a fair chance to fight. Medicines designed for that purpose can have drawbacks, and the indiscriminate suppression of symptoms produced in the fight might be misguided.

But it is a fair question to ask, 'Should you ever suppress the process?' Yes, is the simple answer. From ancient history to now it is agreed and advocated that it is useful in extreme circumstances: modern medicine is at its best in an emergency. If you are run down, have no chance to put your feet up and your body is in danger of being overwhelmed (which, as a parent, feels like most of the time). If you are under attack from something in the environment (a pathogen), then treatment (a drug) may be appropriate.

It is arguable that if you were about to go into the presentation of your career, or Sunday lunch with the new and unsympathetic in-laws, most people would understand you may not want the humiliation of sweating like a pig and coughing up all over the roast.

Short term, in an emergency, once in a while, as a last resort, when my body is losing the battle with an invasion by a pathogen, stopping the system in its tracks is an option we have available in this present world. Hippocrates himself put it perfectly: 'Extreme remedies are very appropriate for extreme diseases.'

I vote for working with my body whenever the problem doesn't fall into any of those more extreme or immediate criteria. Long term I figure I want me and my family to be vigorous, healthy creatures, ready to take on the complex world we live in, our defence systems in tip-top working order. So fit we don't get sick. Generally or too casually, I personally cannot understand why we would want our lovingly evolved, built-in defence system – which has taken aeons to create – to be suppressed. If we discount our 'biological defence mechanisms' as 'symptoms of disease' and treat to suppress them, we misunderstand their very nature, their purpose, their benefits and what they mean about us as humans.

It is the difference between using a dishwasher to clean your plates and smashing them on the ground to solve the washing-up problem.

It has to be understood that the allopathic route is not without consequence. By treating with a substance or procedure intended to halt the symptoms of disease, it can work; but if the body is prevented from dealing with the problem it can have unwanted consequences.

Then a drug is just an umbrella; it keeps the rain off but it doesn't change the weather.

The 'contrary to suffering' principle is aimed at the symptoms. At the level of an invading bacterium (when it would do more harm not to) it may be appropriate to treat with an antibiotic targeted at the bad guys. However, we spend a fortune every year on an ever-growing and probably unnecessary assortment of suppressants, all of which are designed to interfere with our intricate immune systems.

They are not aimed at the pathogen but against our bodies.

Just as an ordinary everyday example, take a common, and seemingly inoffensive, product such as a cough mixture. There are three types. Demulcents, from the Latin to caress soothingly, basically contain syrup, glycerol or honey, and are claimed to reduce irritation by coating the inflamed lining of the airways. Which, as they cannot enter the airways, do no more than coat the back of the throat. Drinking hot lemon and honey will be just as effective.

Then there are opioid derivatives (codeine, dextromorphan and pholcodine) that act directly on the cough centre in the brain, inhibiting the cough reflex. They can stop you coughing in high enough doses by switching off a bit of your brain, but are also likely to cause constipation. And then there are sedative anti-histamines like diphenhyramine; these are popular in cold and flu remedies and work by inhibiting the cough reflex through generally sedating the whole of your brain. They probably work by making you too sleepy to cough. The view of the British National Formulary, the independent drug bible, is that 'the drawback of prescribing cough suppressants is rarely outweighed by the benefits of treatment'.

Judicious use would certainly appear to be wise advice; it seems sensible to be very cautious about whether we use some things at all.

Many other suppressants are designed to stop or inhibit our own natural immune system. They work on our responses; they are not aimed at the bad guys. They work against our 'functions', the bits of us that are essential for us to get through every day. Our functional side is the difference that makes the difference. I accept the 'contrary to suffering' treatment seemed to have done its emergency rescue work on the 'pathology' of Ben's symptoms. His body behaved like it had taken on too much work, with too little or conflicting information and not enough tea breaks. Considering his immune system was so – 'muddled' would be a good word – antibiotic treatment of Ben's infection was probably appropriate.

However, I still have a niggling question: 'What contribution to the problems did we all make with such heavy-handed management of him?' Nineteen hundred years ago, Celsus wrote, 'It makes a great difference, whether a person has been properly or wrongly treated from the beginning, because a method of cure is less successful where it has been applied unsuccessfully.'

Without a doubt, the 'contrary to suffering' principle has had its place in our history, health and survival as a species. It may have brought us – along with good sanitation and improved nutrition – to a time where we now have the luxury to explore beyond emergency treatment. However, 'contrary to suffering' has limitations; it is not good for casual use or when it has to be used for any length of time. It is not great when it is used, not against an invading pathogen, but against how we 'function'. Celsus pointed out that: 'Medicine can do nothing in opposition to nature'.

As we now enjoy a time when we do more than survive, perhaps we can consider what it takes to thrive.

Not everything is an alternative intervention.

Some things do not intervene at all.

*

10. A Paradox or Plausible?

Mungu, the god of all things, and his wife, Mbega, were looking down on the plight of humankind one morning and she asked him if he could help the poor people in their struggles with life.

Mungu replied, 'Gladly, but they are not ready yet.'

At that moment she saw a poor man bowed nearly double by his responsibilities. She was particularly upset by the sight of his ragged sandals that had been repaired many times and which clung to his feet by a few sparse ties of dried, plaited grass.

Mbega turned to her husband. 'Surely you can help this one man?'

Mungu again shook his head and said the man was not ready.

'Shame on you,' she said, 'It would be the easiest thing in the world for you to drop a sack of coins in front of him.'

'Ahh, that is another thing entirely,' said the God of all things.

A vivid bolt of lightening rent the cloudless sky and a sack of the purest quality gold lay on the path in front of the poor man.

Who very carefully lifted his feet so as not to damage his sandals any more and stepped over it, and carried on his weary way.

*

I hate the playground. There, I have said it. Not the school playground (though that one is pretty scary too), no, the one that's all swings and roundabouts. It is always cold, cold and windy. Even in summer it feels cold, probably because it's so bleak. On the one day in the year that it is hot, there is no shade so you are then exposed to relentless sun, smothered in SPF 50 and fighting off the flies. Ours is the most forsaken bit of set-aside half acre rescued from developers. A jigsaw of committee decisions to prevent the rise of gated community, low-maintenance boxes with high-end kitchen appliances in.

Dog poop bins flank the way in and then there is nothing for miles until you hit the 13 allotments tucked under the slip-road from the motorway. All the growing vegetables perfectly absorb the carbon footprint of the traffic. There is a clump of mixed hedgerow the children wee in and then a skateboard park with cctv cameras filming the teenagers who discard used condoms late at night. Somewhere on the circuit the muddle of apparatus springs out of its rubberised patch of land. It is one place I envy the working mums who only see their kids at weekends. After you have stood in it for seven years, you pretty much expect all that primary coloured plastic and metal to entertain your kids for you.

OK, I am not that bad. I will push a bum down a slide and be my fair share of ballast on the see-saw. But the boys are getting heavier and it takes actual effort to get my side down when they both pile on the other end. I will do it, but I insist on another adult to talk to.

All that extra effort that I have to put in these days goes a long way to saving on gym membership. The taller and bulkier the boys grow, the more core strength and biceps I develop and that is how the alternative principle works.

Around about 1964, science came close to cracking the why and how of the like-for-like principle. Just as President Johnson won congressional support to up the stakes in Vietnam and antiwar movements began all over campuses across America, beta blockers were invented. While two cases of typhoid fever in Aberdeen signalled the beginning of the first major food safety incident to occur after the establishment of the NHS, beta blockers became the most widely prescribed drugs for controlling high blood pressure.

Doctors were told never ever to give the drug to patients with congestive heart failure (CHF). As beta blockers work by reducing the heart's pumping capacity, it seemed sensible not to diminish the strength of an already weak heart.

Now, today, most cardiologists agree that beta blockers are the number one drug for CHF.

This is the first time in the history of pharmacology that a class of drug has moved from being forbidden to being the best drug for the disease. Puzzled, square-thinking researchers are searching for an explanation for this phenomenon. Conventional wisdom questions the value of using drugs that make your symptoms worse, in order to make you better in the long run.

This reminds me of a famous story about Mount Kilimanjaro, in East Africa. In 1848, Johann Rebmann, a missionary from Gerlingen in Germany, wrote home about seeing snow on the mountain summit and how his guide spoke of *baridi* ('cold' in Swahili) and how the guide had been to collect the silver from the peaks and returned only with water.

Victorian England rocked with laughter at this 'snow in Africa' story and publicly called the missionary mad. Everything the Victorians knew about the equator ruled out the possibility of frost or freezing temperatures. After all, Rebmann had written this while crossing the arid plains of Tsavo in average temperatures of 85°F. It was an existent fact that equatorial Africa was a land 'where winter never comes'.

Of course, in this lastminute.com world we can book a trip to see for ourselves but, with the resources they had available to them, it was OK for the Victorians to think that. Today, we know the principle of electromagnetic radiation[22] ably explains both tropical heat and freezing temperatures in the same area.

Here we had a drug that works in a way that is 'not possible'. But 'laws of nature' are no more than regularities that have been observed; they are not commandments on tablets. There must be an explanation we just may not know it yet. A pharmacologist at the University of Houston in Texas, Richard Bond PhD, says he has it. He calls it 'paradoxical pharmacology'. Despite it sounding like a contradiction, he believes there is a rational explanation and suspects it lies in an under-explored aspect of the biochemistry of cellular signalling.

It might be easier to imagine that a cell is like a constantly dancing, rhythmically vibrating Koosh ball (those rubbery, syrup smelling, spiky balls you find in pound shops). The outside of a cell, the membrane, is covered with little arms. These are proteins (called receptors), and they are antenna-like parts which act like scanners receiving signals from within our bodies.

Let's say you have a bad heart. After you suffer heart failure, your body pumps out more adrenalin to make your heart work harder. A hormone like adrenalin is an activating signal called an agonist, that binds to the receptor and switches it on. If you are given a drug that mimics the effects of adrenalin, like a shot from cupid, your heart beats harder and you feel better. For a while.

These receptors also respond to molecules called antagonists, which bind to them and prevent them from being activated by things like adrenalin. It would be like putting Sellotape on the fluffy side of Velcro; it stops the hooks being able to fasten on. Lots of drugs are based on synthetic agonists or antagonists that are intended to switch receptors on or off.

As we know, our immune systems (in fact our whole being) seeks balance and, in an attempt to protect from over-stimulation from taking artificial adrenalin for too long, our body starts to switch off its receptors. Which for us, the patient, is a tad inconvenient, as the drug we are taking begins to exaggerate the problem we are taking it for.

However, if you take a beta blocker, initially it is expected that you will get worse and your risk of dying even goes up. But after a couple of months you heart is stronger and studies have shown that health improves and life expectancy rises dramatically. Boom, the like-for-like principle has worked with the body, and balance is restored. A beta blocker called Carvedilol was shown, in 1996, to improve the chances of CHF sufferers living by an amazing 65 per cent. Just to prove a point, not all beta blockers produce this effect, only those that are inverse agonists like Carvedilol. What better description for 'inverse agonism' than like-for-like?

Just like being on the seesaw with children, the more of them you add on one end, the more effort you have to make to get your side down. It kills at first, but it toughens you up after a while.

This isn't the first time 'like-for-like' has made a scientifically verifiable appearance, just a recent one. The principle has triumphed in areas other than tinkering with cell receptors.

The 'law of similars' is a recurring philosophy throughout history, 2,500 years ago, the father of medicine, Hippocrates, said: 'Through the like disease is produced and through the application of the like is cured.' The Delphic Oracle, the shrine to Gaea, Mother Earth, proclaimed: 'That which makes sick shall heal.'

In ancient Jewish writings called Mekhilta (Amharic for 'method' or 'rule'), it says: 'Man does not heal with the same thing with which he wounds, but he wounds with a knife and heals with a plaster. The Holy One, blessed be He, however is not so, but He heals with the very same thing with which he smites.'

Today, hyperactive children are treated with amphetamines (speed), while the skin irritant retinoic acid is used as a treatment for acne. Nobody knows how the drugs work, but your average boffin would expect both to make the situations worse.

Take rhubarb, which has a laxative effect on a well person, has the ability to stop diarrhoea. Senna leaves, used to relieve colic, cause colic in healthy people. The World Health Organisation says Qing Hao (*Artemesia annua*, or sweet wormwood) is the key to fighting the killer fever in the new generation of anti-malarial drugs. It is known to produce the same symptoms as malaria in a person not carrying the protozoa.

After the Japanese scientist Shibasaburo Kitasato (1856–1931) showed it was the toxin that the tetanus microbe produced that made it dangerous to humans, it became a familiar method in the Far East to treat with an antoxin. Meaning 'toxin against toxin', the antoxin is directed against the poison produced by bacteria, not against the bacteria themselves.

In 1901, the first Nobel Prize for Physiology and Medicine was awarded to Dr Emil Adolph von Behring for 'his work on serum therapy against diphtheria'. Behring took the blood serum of an animal cured of diphtheria and used it to cure other animals.

Here is the where the like-for-like principle comes into its own. This work showed antibodies produced by one animal can inform the immune system of another and help to prevent the disease.

This is what came to be called serum therapy, or immunisation.

Taking the principle this one step further and using it, not to cure, but to prevent disease, we end up with probably the world's most successful medical triumph. The overriding success story and the iconic standard of the entire modern medical system has been the immunisation programme.

This is entirely based on the 'like-for-like' principle.

*

By the way, it was a woman who brought immunisation to Britain. The wife of a promising politician, and ambassador on a peace mission to Constantinople in 1716, Lady Mary Montagu. Renowned for her sparkling wit and scandalous poems, she was a society beauty before being struck down by smallpox at the age of 26. Now her face was scarred and her eyelashes had never returned.

Having lost her brother to smallpox two years before, she wrote home from the Turkish city: 'A propos of distempers, I am going to tell you a thing that I am sure will make you wish yourself here.'[23a] She watched old women rubbing smallpox scabs into scratches in people's arms and was assured that no one ever died from the procedure. In March of 1718, Lady M, a woman and an ordinary mother, decided to have her son inoculated.

She was so pleased with the result she declared: 'I am a patriot enough to take pains to bring this useful invention into fashion in England.'[23b] On her return to London three years later, a new epidemic was raging through the city. So Mary's daughter became the first person on English soil ever to be inoculated against any disease.

Here at last, science could deliver on its hopes. This is what science can do for humanity: concrete, testable, repeatable release from suffering. It provides a way to save the human race, literally. As incontestable saviour of the world's health, the rolling out of the immunisation programme has become the cornerstone of modern medicine's delivery on its promise.

Here's the remarkable thing: what we have overlooked is the importance of the principle upon which the success is based. We have gone one step further and used the like-for-like principle not only to cure but to teach the body to handle an invading pathogen better.

It turns out there are not several alternative treatments to 'conventional' medicine, there is just the approach we usually use, and one alternative.

All treatments, modalities, remedies, drugs, herbal teas or whatever your poison is, work in one of two ways: against a problem or with the body. One is a battle against an enemy and another is a civil war. It helps to know if you are fighting a bug, some bad habit of the immune response, or if you are working with the body. The like-for-like principle has a valid place next to the usual route we take.

You can ask your doctor at the handover of the prescription how the drug detailed on the paper actually works. You may be surprised how few people know the answer. However, that is no excuse for not asking. There is always a library, the Internet and, if nothing else, phone the manufacturer. I did all of the above, you call and say 'I am a parent who is being asked to give this to my child. What would you do in my position?' All you want to know is how it works.

One mum questioned the conventions of her time 300 years ago, made an informed decision for her children and changed a nation. I am not saying we all should aim so high, but parents are often best placed to make the links for their own kids. We can make informed decisions (using expert findings) that apply to our children and we can also see clearly when things work. We are the right person, in the right place to make the right decisions for our children, because we know them best.

It turned out one of the anti-histamines Ben was on worked in a way that was not right for him in his circumstance. At least that explained why it had no discernible effect when he took it, but he really enjoyed not suffering the side-effects when we stopped.

And I loved dumping it in the bin.

Neither of the two alternatives, the contrary to suffering or the like-for-like principle, is superior to the other. Both work equally effectively when you use them right. However, like a plaster that you have to put on over cream, if you don't apply it right it won't stick.

Just to go over this again, all treatments fall into one of two groups: working against a bug or working with your body. That's it. The 'contrary to suffering' principle, which stops wild fluctuations, and the 'law of similars' principle, working with the body to achieve equilibrium. If you think of that see-saw in the playground: contrary to suffering is like putting your feet down and stopping the erratic motion so as to bring it to a grinding halt. The 'law of similars' attempts to get the loads even in order to achieve that balance. If another living creature is intent on sucking the life out of you then, just like playing on a playground with the kids, you may occasionally need to stop things in their tracks before they get over-excited and someone gets hurt. But a see-saw is just a plank on a fulcrum if it is not moving up and down. It's meant to rock and it's only fun that way.

The body is always seeking balance and so, in the end neither approach should be dismissed. And more often, a combination of the two works best.

Being aware of the need for balance is the game.

*

You

You can become ill in two ways

with

disease – or – **dysfunction**

you can treat in two ways

either

against the problem – or – **with your body**

11. The Last Toll of the Bell

Modern medicine, as we know it, is less than 100 years old. All the ideas were forming in the dark before the dawning of the scientific age, but it was the discovery of penicillin in 1928, the isolation of cortisone in the thirties, the world's first randomised controlled trials, published in the *British Medical Journal* in 1948, that promised the arrival of a 'provable' saviour of world health. The X-ray taken by Rosalind Franklin that pinned down deoxyribonucleic acid (DNA) in the 1950s, followed by the potential of treat-all 'magic bullets', seemed to guarantee to deliver on the promise.

*

With some things working sometimes when they are not supposed to and others not working when they should, I wanted to know how we got here; in this millennium, treating the way we do. Mostly because it was an excuse not to do housework, I wanted to know why we concentrated on the 'allopathic' path, as opposed to any other approach? Why it is that modern medicine seems oblivious to the like-for-like principle and concentrates on intervention, suppression and management 'contrary to suffering'. I wondered where the point was that this principle took over – if there was one.

I felt that, before our family could move forward, we had to go back. Both approaches to treatment have roots going back of a couple of thousand years ago. Both agree on many things and have similar diagnostic methods. Their foundation of the idea of homeostasis (the body being in balance) has been around since the nineteenth century, and confirmed in laboratories by the whole scientific field of psychoneoroimmunology since the 1970s.

But they have opposite treatment principles.

That is not a bad thing, as both have their uses; the question is why has one taken hold in our culture, when the other seemed just as pragmatic? Or is one of them on the wrong track?

I had learnt about pathology and dysfunction and the real meaning of stress at the physical level of our immune system. From all the work that was done on Ben and Harry, from so many different angles, we had seen both allopathic and the like-for-like principle work – in different contexts.

With all the evidence from modern physics through medical scientific findings to personal experience right in front of me, I wanted to know why the like-for-like was less accepted in our culture. If it was because allopathy had proved such a success, a better method then so be it.

Maybe there really was nothing but snake oil in the like-for-like alternative, a muddle of new-age Adam and Eve beliefs, a naïve story on the periphery of a modern medical system that had succeeded on merit. However flawed, it was possible modern medicine was simply the most effective method of treatment. We are then right to approach life as though treatment is most effective when it interrupts the elegant balance of our existence.

But, imagine if there were another reason for its primacy.

What if its success was just a series of accidental events, many of them not related to medicine at all, that led to it being integrated into our culture?

Imagine if the reason was merely an accident of history.

1,800 year roll back

Timelines were something Ben had started doing in school at this point, so I convinced him my research was helping him with his homework. We pulled out, and dusted off, a couple of those hardback books with cracked spines and the threads showing through. We opened up an Atlas of World History and switched broadband provider to get better download speeds. Slowly we marked history across a line of A4 sheets Sellotaped across the wall above the computer.

It soon became apparent that our medical system really was very new. It has been just over 50 years since the National Health Service was set up, in the middle of an international wave of optimistic fervour over medical science. The NHS vision was to incorporate the very best of the very latest, and the dramatic results of the new laboratories and surgical triumphs overshadowed almost every other form of medicine.

It was not long before this, earlier in the twentieth century, that the profession of the physician actually become respectable. Well into the nineteenth century, doctors commanded little regard, and a little before that there were instances of an 'agreement of cure' – doctors agreed to get you better to a deadline for a fixed fee.[24]

And it has only been 120 years since French chemist and microbiologist Louis Pasteur devised the 'germ theory' of disease. He and his German rival Robert Koch founded medical bacteriology and their work together became the basis of immunisation, which has been with us for no more than three-and-a-half generations.

It wasn't until the end of the nineteenth century that nursing was transformed from a religious calling to a job. The major medical advances – anaesthesia, X-ray and the need for antiseptic/hygienic hospital environments – were all only discovered in the nineteenth century. It wasn't until the Crimean War (1853–06) that we began to understand the role of cleanliness in health.

Two hundred years ago it was still often part of the clergy's job to dance medical attendance when required, and purging, emetics and leeches were the common form of treatment.

About 400 years ago, your grandmother's great grandmother was most likely to have received no more than a blood-letting and a thorough flagellation from a priest to make her feel better.

And that's not long ago.

It does seem that before the collapse of the medieval worldview, the emergence of science and the renaissance, the church had so much influence over scientific progress and there seemed little to learn.

About medicine.

So I went back to the books and turned the pages to Galen, who by now seemed a familiar face, almost a friend. If you look around at what was going on in the world around 200 AD then Galen begins to make sense.

This was a further 1,300 years before modern medical history is usually considered to have begun. And yet Galen's ideas are the foundations of our system; so much so we use his terminology and call our system 'allopathy' after his 'contrary to illness' principle. It is as though the GP surgery door opens directly onto Galen in 200 AD. So that seems a logical place to start excavating the roots of our system.

*

Different books were piling up, with pictures from woodcuts rather than photographs. My kids found it intriguing that surgical procedures were carried out on several people at

116

once, in rooms with columns and moulded ceilings. And the men wore 'dresses'.

I noticed right away that Galen was a reasoning scientist living in a jaded, pagan world that was watching the rise of Christianity. It is the contest between paganism and Christianity that leaves science to jump up and down for attention like an also-ran.

Science, and particularly medicine, was sidelined and even reverted to its superstitious roots. Like a benched player having to watch Christianity doing laps of honour around the whole empire to a cheering crowd. For 1,300 years science, as the Greeks understood it and as we would recognise it, did nothing.

Romans, in general, enjoyed good health. Fully aware of their shortcomings, and in the absence of a full medical knowledge, they embraced what they considered exceptional ideals; prevention, nutrition and good housing, and they understood the role of sanitation for healthy urban living. Remarkably, this resulted in a longevity we are just beginning to see again today.

Romans felt they had complete mastery over the physical world. As Marcus Aurelius remarked 'There is nothing new under the sun', they were even spiritually jaded; men were gods themselves, or emperors were. Gods were dispensable, or at least interchangeable; if you were unhappy with one pagan god, you simply replaced him with another more pleasing to you. They were restless for salvation.

In this kind of atmosphere, the story of Jesus Christ was so compelling that it created hope, an expectation of an eternal life through love of the one God. It drove the conscious evolution of a new culture, and the possibility of harmony with nature, with one another, and with a divine intelligence such as their world had never dreamed.

People began to believe they could transcend their fate. Where philosophy failed to answer why we were here, there flourished an innocent desire for a kingdom of heaven – a kingdom no longer here on earth.

Christianity was considered a compelling reason to ignore further scientific exploration: knowledge which didn't make a man 'wise to salvation' was not only useless, but, more ominously, it was an obstacle on the path to redemption.

So the arena was set for the contest.

On one side you had an indifferent pagan society pursuing knowledge and building up libraries of documented data and on the other you had a fevered evangelical movement whose best idea was that judgment day was coming. A day when everyone would be judged on the purity of their hearts and not how smart they were.

The Circus Maximus

All of which was of course fascinating. But where did Galen come into this and how did he end up affecting our world over and above anyone else – and for so long? He was born in Pergamum and it was here he took up the work that would see him shape the world that was coming. He became a physician to gladiators.

At about the time Galen was 40 he was invited by Aurelius and his co-emperor Lucius Verus to join them in Rome. Here he continued to practise medicine and write and lecture. Not just about medicine but, by keeping 20 scribes on staff, he also wrote prolifically about philology and philosophy. He studied anatomy and physiology and wrote 17 books *On the Use of Parts of the Human Body.* He has around 500 dissertations to his name and his medical writings crystallised and expanded on all the best work of the preceding Greek medical schools and covered nearly every aspect of medical theory and practice of his time.

Galen rightly is one of the greats.

Having read some of his work you understand what an incredible mind he had and the wealth of accurate detail in his writings is astonishing even today. He truly deserves his place in history and in our consciousness today.

But why does his 'contrary to suffering' principle shape much of western medical care today?

To throw a light on this we need to take a look at who Galen was learning from – the gladiators.

*

It wasn't just slaves who were gladiators; criminals were also sentenced to the arena as a means of execution; and even ordinary citizens took it up.

Among Romans, the choice of careers was limited: for most, it was the army, teaching, or the arena. Gladiators, if they were good, earned money and slaves gained their freedom. They were victorious over death or died with great dignity. Displaying the moral qualities that inspired the people, they could be heroes, celebrities, venerated sportsmen and symbols of their empire's dominance and virtue.

If they lived today they would have their own branded clothing line, mobile phone marketing contracts and their pictures in the tabloids.

Back then they were fed three square meals a day and had the right to excellent medical treatment.

This was Galen's area of expertise and he became known as the first sports physician. Frequently found in the bowels of the gladiator pits working on the casualties, he claimed to have 'never lost one under my care'.

It could be here around the gladiatorial arena, the Circus Maximus 1,800 years ago, that the fate of medical progress was decided.

Over the ten days the games usually lasted at that time, the arena was thought of as 'the threshold of the underworld'. Scattered around the amphitheatre were statues of gods like Mars and Diana, and of Hermes, who conducted souls to the afterlife. Men paraded the ground dressed as Mercury, escort of the dead, and Dis Pater, God of the underworld, in a very pagan, carnivalian celebration. The circus was a mocking festival with deity as the warm-up act, a comedian brought in to get the audience going.

The trumpets blared and the grand opening procession began with men carrying ornate chaise longues high over their heads. Known as 'the couches of Libitina, goddess of burials', these were stretchers for the soon-to-be-dead. In the prisons, the gladiators, slaves and criminals, were beaten with rods by staff dressed as demons. Noise filled the stifling dust and heat-drenched air. Swords were scraped sharp on oil-stones, and metal plates and rods lingered in hot coals ready to poke fallen gladiators and check they were really dead. In front of 200,000 spectators there was no faking it.

At the height of its power as a pagan nation, if you called yourself 'Christian' it was heresy against the Roman gods. It was enough to condemn you to a terrible death in the arena. Christians were regularly accused of taking part in crimes like ritual incest, baby-eating and high treason. Rejection of the state religion meant Christians were executed *en masse* to celebrate an anniversary of an emperor's reign, burned at the stake or more often crucified.

At the winter solstice arena games, Christians were the morning's entertainment, to be offered up *ad bestias* (to the beasts). They were made to face wild animals without weapons or armour, a capital punishment ranking alongside crucifixion as the most humiliating of all penalties.

Men with whips forced condemned Christians to face the charge of a lion. Or they were roped to a stake in the centre or rolled out shackled into a miniature chariot as meals on wheels.

It is in this setting that two men, totally unaware of each other, were about to influence the history of Europe forever. One was at the top of his game, the other just getting into his stride.

The first of our 'combatants' was of course Galen. A man with weighted eyes, heavy lids that turned to steel when provoked. He had a nose like the guard on a helmet; it ran straight down from his forehead into his neat moustache and beard. Seemingly always well groomed and calm, he looked like a man who wore a suit of armour underneath his toga. His service under four successive emperors (from Marcus Aurelius to Septimus Severius) coincided with a high point in the triumphs of the Roman Empire, and he was running a huge practice in Rome, with the royal court as his most illustrious clients. On a fiery, controversial quest for intellectual supremacy, he was the leading authority in his field. He had the ear of the emperor, the indulgence of the court and a supply of fresh bodies to study in the arena's casualties.

Up in the gallery, watching the slaughter of criminals, including Christians, was the second player, an African theologian.

Quintus Septimus Florens Tertullianus, from Carthage (now Tunisia), was a man who looked like a hawk. He had round, sharp, swift eyes that noticed the smallest movement and a deeply lined face formed by relentless scrutiny and concentration. He was loosely turbaned, carried a short but unruly beard and wore flowing clothes like a man constantly on the wing.

He watched the Christian slaves in the arena in a ritual intended to degrade and humiliate them and he was deeply touched by the dignity they showed in the face of the taunts, jeering and degradation.[25]

Tertullian became the first theologian to write about Christianity in the language of Latin. This turned out to be the masterstroke Christianity needed to take the game.

The faith may never have survived beyond the Romans had St Paul not preached acceptance of outsiders (Gentiles) in opposition to every other Jewish sect. But it may also have receded back to its Jewish confines had Christianity never been given the winning pass from Latin – this is what enabled Christianity to sweep through Rome and then be carried all over the known world.

This explosion of Christianity is considered to have begun when Tertullian presented a fierce argument for Christians, called the 'Apologeticum', to the provincial governors of the empire in 197 AD. This is an acerbic and dazzling argument for Christianity and a declaration, in the ruling language of Latin, of its absolute superiority. History notes that this fantastic speech, the Apologeticum, gave Christians the means with which to meet paganism on its own ground and defeat it.[26]

Galen had a reputation as the most prolific, cantankerous and effective leading authority on medical thought. Having collated nearly all preceding medical knowledge, he added his own papers and promoted his 'contrary to suffering' tenet as an accepted standard.

By general agreement between writers both ancient and modern, Tertullian was aggressive, sarcastic and brilliant. Combined with writing in the language of power, Latin, he caused Christianity to leap into the mainstream. With Latin propping up the cause, the belief that all there was to know was known, and all there was left to achieve was salvation. So persuasive was the argument, sanctioned by Tertullian, that 'investigation since the Gospel is no longer necessary', all progressive thought stalled in Europe.

The glory that was Greek philosophy and the grandeur that was Rome, mystery cults, oriental and magic, alchemy, astronomy and science, stood on the pitch with the Lord and were overawed.

The new faith took the tournament, in a victory that would influence the next 52 generations. Medical progress was merely one of the casualties of the battle between pagan Rome and Christianity.

Galen was in the right place and time. As the leading player in his field when the whistle went, Galen's vast medical legacy was accepted as total and the general belief was that nothing needed expanding on; it just needed a Christian twist. So Galen's work became the manual that influenced medicine for the next 15 centuries.

The Empire of Christ took Galen's law and wove it so tightly into the fabric of those beliefs that today we can't see it any more. Like a richly embroidered rug, when you are standing on it you only see the pattern and are not aware of the threads that make it up.

The fight back against the Church was not won when Galileo's campaign for 'Copernican heliocentric cosmology' (a sun-centred universe) succeeded or the flat earth was rounded off. It was won when medical science superseded the church as the authority nearest to the heart of the state.

Picture the glorious days, just over 100 years ago, when Pasteur and Koch were finally piecing together the mysteries of the invisible world of germs. Europe must have been in the grip of a feverish excitement, watching scientists pulling stunts with rabid dogs and pens full of anthrax-infected sheep. At a time of great poverty, when housing and sanitation were poor, rickets was common, and life expectancy was around 30 years, breakthroughs into worlds invisible to us must have been a thrill.

The world of microbiology enabled us to see at last what it was that had been troubling us, and the smaller the microbe, the larger the promise of our salvation.

At last we could step beyond mere faith to control our destinies; we had a way to evolve past being victims of the whim of nature.

We invested heavily in the hope of science, we committed emotionally, politically and financially in what was, we believed, our new deliverance. Western medicine sought absolution in science, rushing forward to create the future unable to retrieve the past.

*

Kitale is a Northern Frontier District town near the Ugandan border. It's a well-kept secret by the many who live there, from everybody else who never wants to come anyway. This is where my parents paid two horses and £50 they had to borrow from my grandfather for a patch of poor soil, called it a farm, and coaxed it to yield a life for us.

They poured their sweat and souls into a thousand acres of bush, to build a family out of the dust and dirt-turning and disease that is a farmer's life in Africa. You plough and plant and herd and play the decks with the weather, the bank manager, nomadic herds, plagues of locusts and sickness stacked against you. I didn't know anything else. It was normal. It was simply our life, it was who we were.

I grew up with witchcraft, home remedies like flat coke for stomach upsets, and 'wonder drugs', expensive drugs from a distant, unknown 'home' country. A country I only knew about from Enid Blyton stories, week-old Sunday papers and the World Service. Now I'm here in a leafy-green English garden, reading newspapers that are no longer a week old and drugs are a very ordinary part of our every day and available in the high street. But at some point we lost our home, our livelihood and our life as we knew it – we lost what we were.

Culture shock is about getting used to a different kind of normal.

That sense of dislocation is immense: it is not just about losing a sense of who you are or where you came from; it is about losing any way to remember it.

The foundation of our medical system is rooted somewhere on the other side of a 1,300 year-long void, a religious intermission.

After Galen, medicine's job evolved to endorse theology. There was not much call for anything more. Its greatest use was to patch up the wounded on crusade, disease was divine punishment best purged from you, and death was a release to a better place. After being distracted for so long, the world of western medicine behaved as though it had a profound sense of dislocation from its roots, as though it had lost any way of recovering the centuries of practical experience. Unable to look in a mirror, it had no idea who it was.

Science showed us there was a way we could find ourselves. With its laboratories, technology and techniques of prediction, science promised to by-pass the need for years of practice.

Is it any wonder we grabbed hold of that possibility?

We couldn't go back to get what we had left behind and so rushed headlong toward the future. The pinnacle of our achievements is the programme of immunisation, as the 'provable' saviour of world health it is the legacy of our time.

The immunisation programme is so great it even spells out the rules we left back in 200 AD.

More than a principle method of treatment, it clearly defines the next two rules. Its triumph shows us how staggeringly vital good principles are.

Science works by looking for a pattern to allow us to understand confusion. The more repetitions there are in an experiment, the more it is considered valid. The more repeatable the results, the more weight the proposal gains. Then what tends to happen is the more people who approve of an idea, the more an idea is accepted as right.

Science also expects that if something is 'true' then it is true all the time.

There are no exceptions.

Which is what my family were – an exception.

I guess science is then obligated to look for another pattern to understand the new confusion of an exception. The exceptions within the immunisation programme turn out to lead directly back to forgotten universal rules that make sense of today's problems. They turn a spotlight on ancient principles that make sense in a world searching for a magic bullet.

The immunisation programme taught me the hard way the next rule, which is that the individual is most important.

Not the disease.

The second rule is treat people and not disease.

*

THE 2ND RULE

Treat people, not disease

12. Treat People, Not Disease

A neighbour saw Mwanzi searching for something on the ground.

'What have you lost?' asked the neighbour.

'My cooking stick,' replied Mwanzi. So they both went down on their hands and knees to look for it.

After some time, the neighbour asked:

'Exactly where did you drop it?'

'In my hut,' came the reply.

'Then why are we looking for it out here?' asked the neighbour. 'Ah,' said Mwanzi, 'there's more light out here than inside my hut.'

*

Life began to even out. Ben could eat and he got regular sleep. He had a life at last. The search for a 'cure' turned into a hunt for a cause. If I could find a reason, maybe I would find a better way to help him. You always want to know why, or at least why me?

I was in a bookshop looking for something entirely different, when the owner pushed *A Shot in the Dark* into my hands, a medical history of the pertussis, or whooping cough, vaccination programme. This is the book that led the United States Congress to begin investigation of vaccine-related adverse reactions.

*

Determined that pregnancy will not change anything, let alone stop you going out, you breathe through the birth classes and pick out nursery furniture and paint to match with innocent efficiency. As though becoming a parent is about getting the pregnancy right.

Slowly the problems of raging hormones, bodily changes and status adjustments are heaped on top of hypothetical birth plans and calculations of whether you can cope on a reduced income.

Then in one day, life changes, forever, and suddenly you will receive Mother's Day cards for longer than you have left to give them.

Then the immunisation programme hurtles around the corner before the new parental you can fully emerge from under a mountain of smelly nappies in a stupor of sleep deprivation. You are in no fit state to make a rational or informed decision, or do anything but trust the accepted system and stagger off to a clinic as expected.

Ben's problems escalated in direct connection with his vaccinations (he has only received the DPT – diphtheria, pertussis, tetanus – and polio jabs, so this does not discuss others). We, at least, asked our doctor to talk it through with us and were given a speech about collective responsibility.

'A country is not its geographical location, boundaries or institutions. Or the land-owners or national sports teams. It is the millions of individual people that make up the whole. That "whole" is more important than the individual parts.'

Even though the whole is only the individual parts?

We felt Ben should delay the process.

To his credit, the doctor did say he never went against a parent's instinct. Our failing was that we had nothing more than instinct, a gut feeling, a cautionary family tale to base decisions on.

Nobody heard me, or listened, when I said my sister, Sharon Bernadette Woods, was born on 5 December 1963 and died five months later in reaction to the DPT vaccinations.

Or worse, they dismissed it, saying they couldn't comment on individual cases, but things had changed since then and vaccination was in our best interest.

I didn't know how important those 'individual cases' really are. Medical historian, Harris L. Coulter, and Barbara Loe Fisher, the co-founder and president of the National Vaccine Information Center in America, wrote that seminal book A *Shot in the Dark*. In it they pointed out, 'An impressive number of statements made by vaccine researchers for decades [show] that DPT reactions are "idiosyncratic", ie under genetic control.'[27]

Vaccines have changed in the last 100 years, and even since the Sixties, but genetic predisposition has not. It is the individual who is important in the game of 'facts' conjured from statistics; especially if you are the unlucky individual for whom the consequences toll.

In the future, the Human Genome Diversity Project claims it will be able to profile us into types and make us treatable as individuals. As the evolutionary biologist Richard Dawkins states: 'Hitherto, almost all medical prescribing has assumed that patients are pretty much the same, and every disease has an optimal recommended cure. Doctors of tomorrow will be more like vets in this respect. Doctors only have one species by genotype, but in future they will subdivide that species by genotype, as a vet subdivides his patients by species.' He goes on to point out that 'for some diseases there may be as many different optimal treatments as there are different genotypes.'[28]

Until that happens, you are the only one who can ensure you are treated as an individual.

We were reliant on the way things were – on the way they have always been done. We gave up the question of the individual to the evidence of the population and followed the policy. With facts not readily available to back up our feelings, we caved under the pressure to try the first DPT vaccine and see.

Instinct lost to reason and reasoning.

Ben cried for 36 hours.

The experts (who, by the way, never heard him) considered Ben was simply 'inconsolable', which meant they thought he just would not be comforted (stubborn little thing), and therefore he was dismissible.

Or at least, our 'concern' was dismissed.

But his temperature hardly dropped below 39°C for three days. At the risk of looking stupid again, I phoned the night duty doctor, who told me not to worry.

It was normal.

It was known as the 'triple' when my sister was born and she was given her first jab at just under three months. My parents were told her high temperature was normal, and so were the seizures. After the second jab, her temperature took longer to come down and she had seizures again, only worse. Again, my parents were told this was nothing to be concerned about. Within 24 hours of her third and final DPT shot, Sharon was in a coma.

That morning, Mum went in to get her little baby as usual and Sharon just wasn't there behind her eyes any more. Mum and Dad rushed her to the hospital and were told to wait in the corridor. Their baby and first daughter, my only sibling, was dead by eleven o'clock. All my mum can bring herself to say is that Sharon didn't deserve it.

May she rest in peace.

*

I am the first to appreciate it is not easy to sort out what is just an anecdote or rumour, that has been taken as truth, from hardcore facts that withstand scrutiny. The pertussis vaccine story is a curious and frustrating one of compliance and ignorance. Five decades of physicians, scientists, and government health agencies failing to develop, test and set adequate policy, and drug manufacturers treating the vaccine as a commodity and not monitoring adverse reactions. Added to this is the taboo of discussing its possible re-evaluation.

The reality is that the whole vaccination programme has evolved into a leviathan spanning the globe, advancing over populations and excluding individuals. It has no capacity in its lumbering, lone objective for any one person to be considered in a time-consuming, resource-swallowing, individual way. There is no space for the creative consideration of the single child with a name; there is just the unwieldy single-minded march to herd immunity.

The mass-production mentality is a strong feature of our western culture. This is the mentality that regards the human being not as an individual human but as a product. It is the basis of our medical execution, work environment, education system and religious foundations. It is our habit to lump people all together in a room, treat them, set them tasks, teach them or indoctrinate them and then push them out there as finished products.

This is the way you manufacture sausages, not the way you develop human beings.

When I read *A Shot in the Dark* it was like a light in the night. There was that sense of peace that comes when things make sense. After this, a door opened in my mind and I could see a way out of the hole we were in.

Forty-ish years after my sister was left in a small grave in a small town at the end of a road to nowhere-in-particular in the Third World, the truth (for us) was that nothing has changed.

We are still expected to just turn up. Questions are pre-empted and consent is assumed. Collateral damage is deemed acceptable for the good of the majority, without concrete evidence to that end. And the answers we are given are contained in a public information leaflet left in a waiting room which replies to the question, 'Are there any side effects?' with the words, 'Very few'.

That's it; no details, no information, nothing.

It is one of those things that at first glance seem reassuring, until you think about it. 'Very few' still means 'some'.

All of the following extracts in italics are from 'A Shot in the Dark'.

A pertussis reaction can occur in several stages. First there is an acute or immediate reaction after the injection. This first reaction may be self- contained and followed by a complete recovery. But an acute reaction may also lead to long-term, chronic physical, mental, emotional or neurological disturbances that remain with the child in some form for the remainder of their life.[29a]

They may be considered 'very few' but pertussis reactions can be any number of variations on a theme from a localised red lump to death. They include skin reactions, fever, vomiting and diarrhoea, recurrent coughs, bronchial congestion, ear infections, drowsiness, high-pitched screaming, fretfulness, persistent crying, shock, convulsions, epilepsy, infantile spasms, loss of muscle control, swelling of the brain, blood disorders, diabetes, hypoglycaemia, Sudden Infant Death Syndrome (SIDS) and death.

None of which are denied and all of which are fully documented and a matter of congressional record in America and at the Centers for Disease Control (CDC), and supported in major journals including *The Lancet*, the *British Medical Journal*, *The Medical Journal of Australia* and American journals, and hundreds of books and thousands of articles.

*

Snap your fingers.

A belief can be created that instantly.

But a belief doesn't just exist in that moment; beliefs continue to govern our behaviour and our thinking over time.

It is well documented that we form belief 'strategies', or ways in which we maintain and hold beliefs. Belief strategies are a set of 'evidence procedures' we use to decide whether something is believable or not. Like reality strategies, we hold them in our minds with a consistent pattern of pictures, sounds and feelings. It is precisely because they are so highly patterned that they can last a lifetime.

Biologists say this is fortunate because without these strategies, our understanding of the world and ourselves would not be stable. Our reality, or 'our truth', is our representation of the world; beliefs are the active use of such a map. They help us navigate through each day, whether they are supportive or undermining ones.

The old familiar 'cola conundrum' shows this well.

When testing brain responses to comparing two famous cola brands, neuroimaging experts discovered nothing new. One of the brands wins on blind tasting, but the other sells more.

What caught the public attention were the bits of the brain that lit up under functional magnetic resonance imaging (fMRI). When tasters were blindfolded the region of the brain that responded is called the ventral putamen – the area known to be associated with seeking reward. With no access to other information, more people preferred the taste of one cola, as the decades-old taste challenge adverts claim.

However, when the tasters were told which cola they were drinking, their preferences changed. This time, though, the brain area that showed most activity when using the fMRI was the medial prefrontal cortex – an area known to handle higher cognitive processes. This is the area that is associated with self-referential thinking.

In other words, the choice was then made on what people believed about a brand, their subjective response to it and what they thought that said about them. With an fMRI, you can literally see results that show decisions are often made based on memories, associations and impressions. Rational thought can be as unsubstantiated as emotional reactions. Reality is nothing more than a consensus.

You can talk yourself into any situation using a complex selection of arguments, easily rationalising any decision, and fail to find the courage to investigate your feelings, your gut instinct.

There were so many levels at which we should have considered the question of vaccinations more thoroughly, but the factors are hard to pin down, isolate and prioritise. No matter how enquiring a mind you have, there can seem as if there is no value in questioning when you do not know what questions to ask. There are so many cultural associations wrapped around the subject of immunisation, it can be hard to tell which are yours and which belong to society at large.

The medical profession profoundly believes in what it does; there is no conspiracy. However, in a culture of active promotion and denial of any problems, parents routinely accept that vaccines are safe. Even if you know there are adverse reactions, you rightly believe the statistics show the risk is small and – again – that whatever the risk, it is minimal.

With all the smoke and sleight of hand, we readily focus on the big sell of the small risk.

We believe this to mean that if something goes wrong, it will only be something small. We hardly notice that it actually means the effects could be enormous if you are one of a small number who are at risk.

This is not just about vaccinations.

As new parents, the ones taking the risk with our children, you believe those working in the health support field are well versed in their subject. You believe that in the unfortunate case of there being a problem, you will be supported and sorted out. In addition, you hope that if there were something to question, they would question it, that they know the pitfalls and dangers and the signals to look out for.

You rely on it.

If you voice a concern, you believe they will question the situation if it is something to be concerned about. If they don't, you then assume it is because there is nothing to be concerned about.

Some things are in a grey area, granted. In the case of the DPT immunisation, the connection between allergies, especially milk allergy, and a tendency to react severely to the pertussis vaccine, are complex.

An allergic reaction to a shot is an 'absolute' contraindication (indication against a treatment) to repeated shots, but a pre-existing allergic condition is still an unknown.

However,

As far back as 1953, physicians urged those children with 'allergic diseases' or a family history of allergy, not receive the vaccine.[29b]

This was reiterated again in 1955, 1961 and 1969, and again in 1982.

On my husband's side, he has a life-time history of eczema, asthma and allergies. Ben's background alone should have provoked a red flag-waving, chanting protest in someone's head. Unfortunately, nobody seemed to know any of this. And there they were saying it was 'too complex to understand unless you had the necessary training'.

In my experience, parents (who are the ones who have to take the gamble) are entering libraries and logging-on all over the country, reading medical literature about vaccines and educating themselves and finding the process is easy to comprehend.

Some things are obvious with or without training.

The child who is congenitally vulnerable, had a difficult birth, or had poor health in early life, is a likely candidate for vaccine damage.[29c]

Tick, tick, tick – we had a family history of severe reactions, Ben and I had a long, hard and difficult labour, ending with a ventouse delivery, a meconium birth and his lungs being suctioned, and he had congenital eczema and feeding problems as a baby.

All this time we were being asked whether we had any questions, only to have them treated as a threat. Instead of listening to parents to detect possible problems, it seemed as if the policy was to ally fears at all cost, and then dismiss them with, 'It is known to happen.'

Instead of, 'If it happens, it is an indication for further investigation.'

Just because someone has read the literature and understood there are adverse reactions to a particular vaccine, it is not the same as applying that knowledge practically in the community. Knowing it can happen is not the same as recognising who it can happen to. Knowing something is not the same as knowing what to do with that information.

Those with whom we came into contact were effectively listening to the noise inside their own heads instead of hearing us.

Ben would experience high temperatures for no apparent reason, produce slugs of mucus and not be able to breathe, as though his system had an invisible opposition and went into overkill at the least provocation. He also broke out in such large patches of eczema the health visitors made a house call. Unable to explain them they left, leaving me a book on the subject. Which, I read. It was then Ben began to have this scrambled egg diarrhoea, which he had for months. Although chronic, it was dismissed as toddler tummy.

Histamine causes dilation of the capillaries, constriction of the muscles in the lungs, and increased gastric secretion – all of which are part of the allergic or hypersensitive reaction.[29d]

The eczema became infected and, combined with his diarrhoea, Ben was hospitalised. Where the procedure was wait and be seen for ten minutes by someone who spends that time telling a posse of trainees what you are labelled as. One doctor loudly announced that it was a 'fallacy of coincidental correlation' and not, as he so succinctly added, 'a *post hoc ergo propter hoc*' (after this, therefore because of this). He believed people just thought – wrongly in his opinion – that problems that would have developed anyway were related to immunisations.

It was, in the end, deemed Ben's 'natural' response. So again we were sent home, where it took weeks to treat, which we did with more conventional steroid creams.

Along with leukotrines, histamine is largely responsible for producing much of the reactions seen in asthma, allergic rhinitis, eczema and other allergies.[29e]

We did believe these problems had escalated at the time of his jabs but, like everyone else, Ben was inoculated at three months old, so of course there is no way to tell if he would have been like this anyway.

It is amazing how many things are dismissed as coincidences.

As we have seen, Ben was already vulnerable and, most frustratingly, it may have been exactly his age that fostered a susceptibility.

Data on clinical trials collected together by the British Medical Research Council, included around 50,000 children aged fourteen months or more. Both the US, who never carried out their own tests, and British health authorities have used the trials of the Fifties as evidence that it is safe to give to babies as young as six weeks.[29f]

Yet, the axiom is the lower the weight, the lower the dose.

On a bottle of cough mixture there are instructions for smaller doses to be given to smaller people. Yet a two-month-old baby receives the same amount of vaccine as a 14-

month-old who weighs three times as much and has an immune system robust enough to cope with kindergarten.

By the way,

the level of reaction in those trials was 42 babies who experienced convulsions within 28 days, which translates a high one in 1,000 children. Convulsions were the only noted reaction; no others were taken into account, so this does not even reflect the true height of the potential reactions.[29g]

We had several discussions with the health service and settled on not dropping out, but not proceeding with the course until Ben was two. When I say 'discussions' I mean letters through the post, summons to the surgery, being pulled aside at every health check for a 'chat', personal calls to our front door and mild threats.

I had to ask: 'With my family history what would you do?'

We and Ben muddled along for a year and a half, and, true to our decision, finished the course. We fulfilled our part of the bargain and he had the final two shots.

I now believed Ben's immune system should be strong enough to take the dose as advised. However, I had missed the fact that subsequent shots are given only to solve the problem of poor antibody response in newborns and are not an essential or an obligatory part of an effective inoculation process.

Moreover, the affects are accumulative. Like doing housework without Marigolds is bad for your nails. When your hands are constantly in water – unlike your skin, which can unprune itself – nails can't repair themselves between chores.

He was now old enough to voice his discomfort. After the second shot, the first of these vaccinations, he wailed and complained about a headache and the leg into which he was injected became stiff and tender, recovering slowly over a week.

British health officials have considered a severe local reaction to be a contraindication to further injections of pertussis vaccine. All local reactions should be reported to the doctor who administered the shot, and he should not dismiss the reaction lightly.[29h]

I asked about proceeding and was told this was normal. The notes from two years earlier were probably overlooked and I'm sure we didn't repeat everything to everyone, because there were so many people involved. Hoping to bump into one person who has an overall picture, it is easy to forget people defend what they believe in and our brains work to make the world fit the picture. You are the only one with your story and the only one who can make any sense of it all.

After the third and final jab, his reaction was a subtle behavioural and cognitive meltdown into quiet chaos. Although he appeared ordinary to everyone else, we watched him lose concentration as he struggled to hold a steady picture of the world. He was hyperactive, had a short attention span and became a 'muddlehead'.

Far from 'hot-housing' Ben, I had been struggling to keep up with his productive curiosity. After the shots, he never seemed quite with it. You could see him in the middle of his school show wondering what the audience was doing there.

There is evidence the B.pertussis toxin, whether it enters a body through the vaccine or via the disease, can cause a variety of neurological damage ranging

142

*from the profound to the more subtle forms – asthma,
learning disabilities, hyperactivity, attention span and
behavioural disorders or chronic earache for
example.*[29i]

Ben developed into an oddball with so many quirks, like
most of us I wondered if I was missing something huge, I
even thought of Asberger's syndrome (a form of autism). But
somewhere in there was a bright child struggling to put the
connections back together.

It is well documented that children with allergies
experience constant discomfort in their skull cavity; they
often display symptoms of withdrawal or 'disengagement'.
He was not disabled, just unable to be normal. His favourite
toy was the inside of his head. He was imprisoned in that
space, the difficulty of communicating with reality too hard
a struggle to keep up.

It was easier to play inside his head than try to hear
through muffled ears and see through stinging eyes, and he
could not taste or smell anything. For him, a head full of
pain was normal, for me the only normal thing about him
was his Buzz Lightyear obsession.

He wore his Buzz PJs every day and would only answer
if referred to as Buzz. While he was wearing 'the uniform',
he was on duty. He could only stop zooming round the
galaxy encountering aliens and fighting off Zurg if he put a
jumper over the top. He couldn't just stop; he actually had
to be 'turned off'.

I didn't realise he was in fact under attack from unseen
enemies the rest of us didn't share.

*A child with allergies has a hypersensitive immune
system; one that is ready to react instantaneously to
contact with any allergenic substance ... it stimulates*

a violent reaction that is intensified by the presence of histamine. Any substance that increases the production of histamine, or exaggerates the body's sensitivity to it, will intensify an allergic reaction.[29j]

I suspected – no, I was sure of – the connection to the vaccines, but everyone denied it and we were made to feel hysterical. I know that just because the majority of people believe something does not make it true, but we only had our experience with no facts to back up, what seemed at best a tenuous argument.

Another name for the pertussis toxin is HSF, or 'Histamine Sensitizing Factor', meaning that it increases the body's sensitivity to the action of histamine. It switches on this sensitivity to histamine, making any allergic reaction intense and aggressive.[29k]

He was the kid who reacted like he had flu to every cold, constantly ill, struggling to make head or tail of what the rest of us take for granted. The diarrhoea eventually became yellow and foamy, like diluted cavity-wall insulation.

The pertussis toxin is also known to stimulate the production of a catchy little thing called IgE, an antibody that mediates the allergic response. An allergic condition is characterised by an increase in levels of IgE. Many physicians and scientists have noted the relationship between allergy in a child and a severe pertussis vaccine reaction.[29l]

*

There was no easy-to-trace, convenient, linear cause and effect. It isn't always a question of the big picture or right or wrong, of throwing out, or shunning a whole idea. It is not about sides or competing arguments. It is an internal struggle to assess your place in the demographics and statistics; a challenge to balance competing ethical claims, where sometimes it is easier to understand the position of the other side.

I understood the desire to protect ourselves from diseases that once took countless lives. I understood the benefit/risk ratio. I understood the community responsibility. I understood the absolute belief in the virtue of vaccinations.

But it is only faith that doesn't question.

Being afraid to ask questions leaves the unsaid to become assumption. My sister's death was a no-go area; I grew up understanding it hurt my mother and father to talk about it and so I believed that it was better not to. We never spoke about her during all of Ben's problems or even after all this happened; until this search for answers. Had I asked them questions all this may have been avoided.

To dare to question any convictions sharpens our focus and breaks the cycle of conditioning. It sorts out what is relevant to you now, today, and what is inherited, half learned and just plain accepted without question. It gives us the opportunity to come out of any life-debilitating trance we may be caught in.

Any belief we hold, from believing spiders are dangerous to believing the kids will learn to tidy their own rooms one day, is created by us to protect us. According to psychologists, biologists and neuroimaging brain-mappers, we do not hold a belief if it does not in some way protect a core value, and we have a value attached to every belief held. To change them is to challenge the supporting columns of our minds. To shake the foundations of our being and rebuild the world as we know it.

*

Ben was standing on a chair one morning, arms spread out and muttering things about coming to the rescue. As I past him with a pile of ironing, I asked him if he was pretending to be Buzz Lightyear and he replied: 'No mummy, I am Buzz Lightyear. Sometimes I pretend to be Ben.'

*

There is no easy answer, however much we want to imagine a simple formula to be enough to storm the gates of heaven. However much it would be nice to have a simple set of beliefs or activities we can rely on and concentrate on, the only result of this is conditioning.

The vast majority of people fall within the statistically safe boundaries; the trick is to determine if your children do. Then you can protect them with the best option and – again – for the vast majority this is through immunisation.

For Ben, though, the truth was that he now found it easier to be a fantasy superhero and less comfortable to be a normal child in the real world. He was three-and-a-half and trapped inside a body that was constantly fighting itself in a world of benign matter that had turned hostile.

Arguably our greatest modern success, the global immunisation or vaccination programme, along with clean water, can be argued to have made the most significant contribution to the health of our species. However, we are now in the luxurious position of being able to refine the protection of all our children in a way that is more individual.

Its failings teach us The 2nd Rule.

The universal principle that the immunisation programme has to teach us is that no matter how effective a technique is, it depends for that effectiveness on the individual being treated. Some 20 centuries ago in ancient India, Charaka, a noted practitioner of Ayurveda, said in his famous Ayurvedic treatise Charaka Samahita, 'A physician who fails to enter the body of a patient with the lamp of knowledge and understanding can never treat diseases. He should first study all the factors, including environment, which influence a patient's disease, and then prescribe treatment.'

It is people that we treat, not diseases.

It is our individuality that matters, that is the difference that makes the difference.

*

13. Ask Now and Shoot Later

Eight questions you need to answer.

1. Is my child sick right now?

2. Has my child had a bad reaction to a vaccination before?

3. Does my child have a personal or family history of:
   – vaccine reactions
   – convulsions or neurological disorders
   – severe allergies and/or eczema
   – immune system disorders

4. Do I know if my child is at a high risk of reacting?

5. Do I know how to identify a vaccine reaction?

6. Do I know what to do if there are any reactions?

7. Do I know how to report a vaccine reaction?

8. Do I know I have a choice?

(Provided by the National Vaccine Information Center www.909shot.com)

The National Vaccine Information Center (NVIC) is a non-profit educational organisation founded in 1982. Located in Vienna, Virginia. NVIC is the oldest and largest parent-led organisation advocating reformation of the mass vaccination system and is responsible for launching the vaccine safety movement in America in the early 1980s.

It is a comprehensive and informative, award-winning organisation with a user-friendly site.

www.immunisation.nhs.uk is the official NHS site and is clear and functional. You will find the advice is general with the reminder that any individual concerns must be dealt with at the time with the nurse.

It is understandable that the services are very careful not to answer specific questions about vaccination and state clearly that you should see the experts, the doctor or nurse, dealing directly with you.

But remember, you too are an expert – in your child.

Nobody else is.

We as parents would do well to remember that a vaccine doesn't come with a guarantee. It doesn't work every time or last forever, and it's not a case of one size fits all; because we are individuals, the response will not be uniform. When, or if, you immunise your children, remember to approach it as the start of a process and not an event at the clinic which you then walk away from. It is important to remember your child needs caring for in the same way as if they are sick; give their bodies the nurture you would to get them well.

Even if they seem fine.

A pain of any kind is a body trying to communicate.

Make sure their immune system is not compromised in any way at the time. Remember: an over-loaded immune system has a harder time doing its job and recovering, too.

Bring up any fears you have, any concerns, any questions at all and keep doing that until you feel someone has listened. Do not be afraid to be stupid. Go ahead only when you feel satisfied with the answers you have been given; make sure they are relevant to you and not generic. Don't expect them all to come from the clinic. You can walk away at any time and return later.

The relationship is one of a consumer and a retailer, each with their own agendas. Health professionals are manufacturers, warehousers, buyers and purveyors of fine goods, selling something they are utterly convinced you should have. Because they believe in the product, doesn't mean it is right for you or that you want it. As it is we who bear the consequences, it is we – the parents – who need to be better informed. It should be our responsibility to decide and, as such, it is then the responsibility of those who hold the information to be clear and concise and forthcoming with it.

The immunisation programme is, arguably, the most successful medical advance in the world, and as such, a supportable technique. Not only because it can statistically prove to be effective, it adheres to the 'like-for-like' principle of working with the body, treats like-for-like working with the body's functions, and holds up all four rules.

In the end, it comes down to you to bear the consequences of your decisions, so find out what is true for you.

*

- Vaccines may cause problems for people with certain allergies. For example, people who are allergic to the antibiotics neomycin or polymyxin B should not take rubella vaccine, measles vaccine, mumps vaccine, or the combined measles-mumps-rubella (MMR) vaccine.

- Patients who are allergic to antibiotics such as gentamicin sulphate, streptomycin sulphate, or other aminoglycosides should check with their physicians before taking the influenza vaccine as some influenza vaccines contain these drugs.

- Anyone who has had a severe allergic reaction to baker's yeast should not take the hepatitis B vaccine.

- People with certain other medical conditions should be cautious about taking vaccines. Influenza vaccine, for example, may reactivate Guillain-Barré syndrome in people who have had it before. This vaccine may also worsen illnesses that involve the lungs, such as bronchitis or pneumonia.

- People who have had Guillain-Barré syndrome, or neurological disorders, should not receive the DTaP vaccine.

- Some vaccines, including those for influenza, measles, and mumps, are grown in the fluids of chick embryos and should not be taken by people who are allergic to eggs.

- Vaccines that cause fever as a side effect may trigger seizures in people who have a history of seizures related to fever.

- Certain vaccines are not recommended for use during pregnancy.

- Women should avoid becoming pregnant for three months after taking the rubella vaccine, measles vaccine, mumps vaccine, or the combined measles-mumps-rubella (MMR) vaccine as these could cause problems in the unborn baby.

◆ Women who are breastfeeding should check with their physicians before taking any vaccine.

◆ In general, anyone who has had an unusual reaction to a vaccine in the past should let their physician know before taking the same kind of vaccine again.

◆ The physician should also be told about any allergies to foods, medicines, preservatives, or other substances, and if there is a compromised immune system caused by anything from HIV to a cold.

(Source: *The Gale Encyclopedia of Nursing and Allied Health* and the *CDC Guide to Contraindications to Vaccinations*)

Internet Information

In the world with a super highway there are so many roadside stops, it is not always easy to know where to pull off. Like a good travel guide here are some recommendations. They are the personal opinion of the writer but, they are highly reputable, 5-star choices, so hardly difficult to endorse.

Centers for Disease Control National Immunization Program, www.cdc.gov/vaccines/

Global Alliance for Vaccines and Immunization (GAVI), www.gavialliance.org/

National Vaccine Injury Compensation Program, www.bhpr.hrsa.gov/vicp

An award winning independent web resource, www.healthline.com

Immunization Action Coalition, www.immunize.org/

From the Immunization Action Coalition; vaccine information for the public and health professionals, www.vaccineinformation.org

THE 3RD RULE

Prevention is better than cure

14. Prevention is Better Than Cure

Just over 200 years ago, a report, by William Thomas, the Sanitary Inspector for the district of New York, rated the city among the worst in the world. He wrote, 'Filth of every kind thrown into the streets, covering their surface, filling the gutters, obstructing the sewer culverts, and sending forth perennial emanations which must generate pestiferous diseases.'

The commercial avenues of the area were paved with cobblestones, between which refuse collected and rotted. The streets were 'very filthy' with accumulations of manure from horses and, in winter, the dead dogs, cats and rats, household and vegetable refuse accumulated to depths of three feet or more. 'Garbage boxes', rarely emptied, overflowed with offal, animal carcasses, and household waste. While poorly designed sewers had been installed throughout the region, pools of stagnant water collected over sewer drains that were generally clogged. Most of the population depended upon the outdoor 'water closets', close to wells used for drinking. The few amenities that were provided were generally inadequate, often becoming public health hazards themselves.[30]

*

When I was pregnant, both times, I became an addict. Not in any Class-A drug way, but through a compulsion for catalogues. I wasn't mugging old ladies for their bus money to support the habit, but I just could not stop putting myself on mailing lists and leafing through classified ads looking for more of them.

The whole thing – having babies – taps into a deep paranoia. How will the poor little, helpless, thing ever survive? It is not enough that billions have done so since we walked out of Africa; the argument goes something like: 'Well, none of them had me for a mum.'

How will my baby survive me?

If I had to go to classes to learn to breathe, when that was something I thought I had been doing for a long time, what else was I missing?

A lot – it seems – is necessary for the survival of all babies. Not just big stuff like good food, clean bottoms and at least two hour-stretches of sleep, but so many little things from door jams and potty-training stickers to nickel-free poppers on organic-cotton sleepsuits.

How does any child ever get to seven without all this stuff?

I know I am not the worst sufferer, and I have kitchen cupboard door-locks in the back of the cupboard still unused, and something in the loft that was supposed to go in the car to hold everything I might need for travelling. If it had Satnav it might have had an edge, but it actually only doubled up on the ordinary change-bag and it has never left the house.

Stair-gates at least made sense, or at least made it possible to finish a cup of tea sitting down. Whenever I took my babies anywhere that had open stairs that is where you would find me. At the bottom of them, pretending to love their game of trying to crawl up as far as possible before inevitably falling down. Those were the fun days.

Danger lurks around every corner of a table if those catalogues are anything to go by, so every pregnancy turns into a prevention marathon; a mad dash to think of every conceivable thing that could go wrong and stop it happening.

Vaccinations are like stair-gates, a better thing to have than the rush to emergency to stem the blood spurting from a two-inch deep gash in the temple. According to the Centers for Disease Control and Prevention, National Immunization Program statistics from the developing world show that more than two million people a year, mostly children, die from vaccine-preventable diseases. In developed countries when immunisation rates fall, diseases reappear. Vaccines are remarkably safe and effective. In America, each one undergoes about ten years of research before the FDA approves it.

This is the third fundamental rule that the vaccination programme has to teach us: prevention is better than cure.

We owe it all to cows.

Mad cows and royalty, really.

Taken from the Latin word for cow, *vacca*, it all began in the fields of rural eighteenth century England, when farmers and country physicians told stories of milkmaids who contracted cowpox from cows and then tended not to get smallpox. A young Gloucestershire country doctor, Edward Jenner (1749–1823), having had success with smallpox inoculation, became obsessed with this connection; that a minor disease in cows had the possibility to free people from one of the great scourges of human health.

Cowpox, to cows, is a relatively minor infection of the udder, leading to a slight decrease in milk production. It can also lead to a case of pox in humans that might scar, but not nearly to the extent of smallpox, and it is not fatal.

An outbreak of cowpox in 1796 allowed him to experiment. He extracted fluid from an oozing pustule on the hand of Sarah Nelmes, a milkmaid who had cowpox. He used it to inoculate eight-year-old James Phipps who went on to prove resistant to smallpox also.

Warned against publishing his paper anywhere out of concern for his reputation, Jenner struggled for 25 years to persuade the medical establishment of the benefits of his new technique. Only when it was accepted and supported by the royal families of Europe, did the English parliament pass a law in 1840 making it compulsory.

A notion leapt out of mundane folklore into law.

It has since grown to be a public health intervention with one of the greatest impacts on the world's health. Over the following 100 years, two more vaccinations were introduced: rabies and the plague. Since the introduction of the diphtheria vaccine in 1923, nine major, global diseases have been added to the list. More minor ones are added regularly. Although the first vaccines are, in some respects, crude, vaccines in general have contributed dramatically to reducing the death rates from disease.

On a grand scale, vaccination is credited as the practice that enabled science to replace the church at the heart of State. It is the only true medical prevention technique: unlike early diagnosis and treatment, or preventative surgery, it is the only technique that works with the body before it is diseased – and improves its performance.

Vaccination is considered a valid, repeatable programme that is accepted as vital, yet – again – its shortcomings can teach us the full meaning of the principle of prevention. It is not the only reason we are enjoying the longest life expectancy since Roman times.

Despite the growth of medical knowledge in eighteenth century Europe, the general health of the population slowly deteriorated as more people moved to dirty, crowded, industrialised cities and standards of public hygiene declined.

Without clean water, sanitation, improved nutrition, and better housing we would still live knee-deep in effluent and there is no inoculation for that.

Like a home safety kit full of plastic cupboard latches, fold-out toilet sets, and desalination tablets, prevention – in all guises – falls into the category of being better than a cure.

Hippocrates pointed out the role of a good diet, fresh air and cleanliness as being better than cure. Charaka said: 'It is more important to prevent the occurrence of disease than to seek a cure.' Seven hundred years ago Paracelsus laid out the principle in medieval writings. Two hundred years ago, along with all of the above, even changing the bed linen was prescribed as a preventative technique.

In many communities in Africa, where sanitary conditions are poor and there is little or no effective use of hygiene as a prevention method, the World Health Organisation estimates that 1.5 million children die each year just from whooping cough. Contrast this with us here in the West, who enjoy better housing and clean environments, and where the sun never sets on fully-stocked supermarkets. Simple habits like washing hands and wiping hard surfaces can help prevent whooping cough infection, which is transmitted by contact.

It is easy to be convinced that the life-saver is the safety-catch on the oven door, when really it is in learning not to touch hot things.

Considered one of the most radical, political and social thinkers in the second half of the twentieth century, Ivan Illich has written exhaustively about the effects of improved housing, sanitation and diet on the decline of infectious diseases. He said that: 'sanitation, inoculation and vector control, well-distributed health education, healthy architecture, and safe machinery' have the greatest effect on health. And, he added, especially if they are supported by a 'truly modern culture that fostered self care and autonomy'.[31]

If you offer a pill to a man to cure his repeated bouts of malaria, he is likely to think you are a miracle worker and the secret is in the pill.

Without your pill he is helpless.

Yet malaria is a preventable disease.

It kills more than one million people a year, 90 per cent of them in Africa – mostly children – and the most effective way to deal with it is not to get it.

Prevention is very easy; all it takes is a little knowledge.

Covering open water with a layer of oil will prevent malarial mosquitoes laying eggs. Knowing the lifecycle of the female mosquito tells you what time of day to be cautious. Rubbing certain scents on your skin (such as citronella) to repel mosquitoes, and – proved to be most successful – sleeping under nets at night keeps the pests at bay. All of which are cheap, effective, everyday, simple, lifestyle changes that can prevent malaria.

Epidemiological evidence shows that, 18 years after compulsory vaccination was introduced and four years after a strict drive to vaccinate the population achieved a 97.5 per cent success rate, England experienced the worst smallpox epidemic between 1870 and 1872. Forty-four thousand people died, three times as many as during an earlier epidemic when fewer were vaccinated.

After the high incidence of smallpox and related deaths proved vaccination didn't work as effectively as thought, the town of Leicester relied entirely on improved sanitation and quarantines during the 1872 epidemic. The town had 19 cases and one death per 100,000 population, whereas a comparable Warrington had six times the number of cases and 11 times the death rate of Leicester, even though 99 per cent of its population had been vaccinated.[32]

The vaccination programme teaches that prevention is better than cure. However, when even housework is a preventative measure, it would seem that there is more to prevention than vaccination.

*

But, again, it is vaccination that can teach us the ultimate definition of prevention. We give a vaccination to teach the immune system, not to prevent disease – this is a very important distinction.

Vaccinations and medications don't really protect people; it is our immune systems that protect us and keep us safe. A stair-gate, though a pretty good thing to prevent children from accidentally falling down, is no substitute for learning to climb steps.

It is our immune system that is the ultimate prevention measure.

Louis Pasteur regarded Claude Bernard as 'Physiology Itself', even though Bernard had contradicted Pasteur's claim that germs cause disease. Even after Robert Koch designed an experimental procedure – now called Koch's Postulates – Bernard still could not help pointing out the flaw in the idea of 'the germ theory of disease'.

To prove that germs were not the cause of disease but would – and could only – thrive if an ideal environment for them already existed, Bernard pulled a great stunt in a room full of physicians and scientists. Taking a large glass of water infected with cholera he turned to his colleagues and declared: 'The germ is nothing and the terrain is everything,' before draining the glass like an alcoholic falling off the wagon.

He never contracted the disease.

There was a famous German pathologist, Rudolph Virchow (1821–1902), who said: 'Germs seek their natural habitat – diseased tissue – rather than being the cause of the diseased tissue,' and compared it to mosquitoes that seek stagnant water, but do not cause the water to become stagnant.

Our bodies are the terrain; if the blood, body fluids, tissues, cellular functions, etc., are in balance, a 'terrain' is created that does not support the life of a disease.

In the same way that glass is a slow moving liquid, it turns out that our blood proves to be a mobile tissue and, for a long time, many researchers and doctors believed, and plenty still do, that blood is sterile.

This is not surprising, as blood tests offered in most practices today consist of the standard methods of using stains or electron microscopes. Both processes are limited in that the blood is effectively killed through the processes used in observation.

Looking at a lump of cheese does not tell you much about milk.

The serum of every human being, and warm-blooded animal, is busy with foreign life forms. These can be seen with Darkfield Microscopy (a high-calibre microscope with a super-fine resolution, which uses a dark background with light reflecting the object from the side to enable the smallest of living forms to be observed). A professor Dr Gunter Enderlein (1872–1968), zoologist and entomologist, microbiologist and researcher, called these life forms *endobionts*, from the Greek 'endon' meaning internal and 'bios' meaning life. He figured out how important the 'terrain' was by watching these tiny little critters and how they thrived or died.

They flourish in a strong alkaline pH environment without causing disease. As your blood becomes more acidic you become more accommodating to bacteria. If you become only a little more acidic, fungal life forms enjoy the climate, and finally viral forms are attracted to, and succeed in, a strong acid pH. The more acidic the pH value of our body, the more accommodating we are to the wrong company.

The germ theory cannot account for the fact that if you expose 100 people in a school hall, all breathing – sharing – the ever-circulating air, full of rampant pathogens, that there will be individuals in that room who do not develop that season's bug.

Nothing is a substitute for robust health as a preventative measure.

There are seven effective prevention methods, in order of priority:

- A strong, well-supported, immune system.
- Clean water.
- Good nutrition.
- Sanitation and personal hygiene.
- Exercise.
- Vaccination.
- Healthy housing.

To make 'prevention' as a practice even a little exciting you may have to hoover in the nude, but all these methods are effective and simple: and better than the alternative – being ill. Thanks to these measures, we are less often exposed to disease and better able to withstand it when we are exposed.

*

That is not the end of the story; life is not all about fighting disease; oh no, no, no. . . it's worse. Diseases are the least of our problems here in our developed world. Now that we have bugs disinfected, sterilised, pasteurised and demoralised we are left surviving more or less into old age. No longer under attack on a daily basis, we are left noticing that our bodies take a battering in other ways: we are becoming aware of the toll taken by normal daily life. Less than five per cent of illness in the developed world is pathogen based; the biggest killers in the West are chronic, dysfunctional illness and degenerative diseases of old age.

Again, prevention is better than the alternative. A healthy body is not just a defence against other species trying to kill us, it is also a defence against, or postpones for many years, chronic and degenerative illness.

A full 80 per cent of illness is preventable.

According to the World Health Organisation, tobacco is the largest, single, preventable cause of cancer. Raised blood pressure causes strokes and heart disease. There is a causal link between alcohol and more than 60 types of degenerative disease. A high cholesterol level increases the risk of coronary heart disease. By 2015, 700 million adults will be obese and 7.4 per cent of the population will die from it. Low fruit and vegetable consumption is a risk factor for cancer and cardiovascular disease. Physical inactivity will kill two million of us a year and 3.3 per cent of us will die from illicit drugs, unsafe sex or iron deficiency – all preventable.

In fact, a study, begun in 1965, found over the next decade that the healthiest people followed seven common preventative measures. These made the most difference to long-term, overall health and resulted in preventing or postponing the largest threats to our modern lives: chronic, degenerative and dysfunctional illness. The seven healthiest, happy habits of the longest living are:

- Sleeping seven to eight hours a night.
- Eating properly.
- Maintaining a reasonable weight.
- Not smoking.
- Drinking alcohol in moderation.
- Taking part in some sort of physical activity.
- Having numerous connections to friends.

Each practice alone contributed to better health, and the combined effect of all of them gave people bodies 30 years younger in tests compared to those who followed less than three of these habits.

Now that's sexy.

Stay healthy, and look younger, without surgery.

I never worked out if those safety things that keep fridge doors shut were for the kid's sake, or to stop us from comfort-eating our way through their tantrums.

Because some of what we do doesn't seem relevant there is no reason to think we can do without it. And we don't have to think 'this is as good as it gets', depend on medical care and accept a slow degeneration into chronic disease. Nobody suggested that New Yorkers, or their European counterparts, should go back to living in caves. Instead, following a report by the Council of Hygiene of the Citizen's Association in 1867 – when Manhattan contained some 15,000 tenement houses – the first tenement house law was passed. Now we all have drains, rubbish collections and 100 per cent germ-destroying household cleaners.

We have a wealth of complex natural drugs on call, in the right dose, delivered accurately, and withdrawn without side-effects just as successfully, but with support, our immune systems can do more than pull us out of the mire. A proper respect for our immune systems will go a long way to preventing not only disease, but long-term degenerative conditions which, arguably, we should be more afraid of. A healthy immune system is the most effective prevention measure, not only against disease now but against degenerative diseases that could be ahead.

In a world where nothing is guaranteed, as well as taking advantage of the immunisation programme, we parents can ultimately *keep* our children well, and 'future insure' their health. Most effectively through simple preventative measures such as good nutrition, proper rest, running around and most importantly having fun.

*

Heuristic techniques use readily accessible, though loosely applicable, information to problem-solve. You can use these techniques to make decisions, come to judgments, and solve questions, especially when facing complex problems or when you have incomplete information.

If you are having difficulty understanding a problem ...

1. Try drawing a picture.

2. Choose other words to describe your problem, another definition could open up another solution.

3. If the problem is abstract, try examining a concrete example.

4. Find a similar problem you have solved and see if you can apply the solution from that problem.

5. Assume that you have a solution and 'work backward'.

6. Go through the assumptions you have and challenge them.

7. Try solving a more general problem first, a more ambitious plan may have more chances of success.

8. Remove variables to simplify the problem.

9. When one approach fails, try the opposite.

Much of the work of discovering heuristics in human decision-makers was ignited by cognitive psychologists, Amos Tversky, Daniel Kahneman and Gerd Gigerenzer.

15. Where Do You Keep the Bananas?

‘The constancy of the internal environment is the condition that life should be free and independent. So, far from the higher animal being indifferent to the external world, it is on the contrary in a precise and informed relation with it, in such a way that its equilibrium results from a continuous and delicate compensation, established as by the most sensitive of balances.’

Claude Bernard, French Physicist, 1813–78

*

One of my boys loves bananas, and one hates them. I think bananas are funny. It's a funny word, in a way that 'bread' is not funny. Harry's favourite joke is a banana joke he made up: 'Why did the banana bump into the wall?' Obviously the punch line is not funny; he was four when he thought it up. But here it is: 'Because it didn't look where it was going.'

Actually, I put my hands up, I do think it is hilarious. The word banana will now always remind me of the day he told that joke. It takes me back to the room, I know how old he was, I can see his face creasing up right now. I can't help but smile just at the thought.

In fact, the word 'banana' conjures up a whole collection of memories. Comic strips from the *Beano*, a Woody Allen movie, a Velvet Underground album cover, large ones in blue pyjamas. Memories of rubbing the inside of the skin on insect bites to reduce the swelling and irritation. Of Uganda, where their word for banana is the same as the word for food.

Just the word conjures up recipes, times I have bought bananas and I can even remember actual bananas I've eaten. Yet there is no box or storage unit, that exists somewhere definite, that keeps this word for us to use when we want it.

Nevertheless, the memory, and the physical recall of it, is very real; just the word triggers genuine cellular reactions. I can actually smell a fresh, yellow one or an old brown one just by thinking about them. The taste and texture, how the strings feel if you bite into one you didn't peel carefully. Information is separate from our physical form and yet we actually salivate just at the memory of a banana; physical reactions to nothing but a thought, as brain cells don't contain any actual 'banana'.

The same thought can trigger the same physical reaction every time even though the atoms in your body come and go all the time, when in fact 98 per cent of your body was not here a year ago.

The configuration of cells remains roughly constant, but atoms pass back and forth through cell walls and so every three months you have a new skeleton. Every six weeks you have a new liver. You have a new skin every month, which is why tans fade. Every four days you have a new stomach lining, and the cells that make contact with your food are being renewed every five minutes. Even the atoms in you brain come and go; the content of carbon, nitrogen, oxygen and so on is totally different as you read this than it was a year ago.

Yet we are still physically here and the word 'banana' and all that it means for us does not disappear. We can pluck it out of the air.

The structure of human physiology has been studied in great detail and has been pinned down to a twisted ladder of sugar and phosphate molecules, with 'rungs' made of nitrogen-containing chemicals called nucleotide bases. This very thin string chemical – a one foot long string of normally squeezed into a space roughly equal to a cube one-millionth of an inch – is called DNA.

DNA is the blueprint, referred to as a gene, for every protein. Every one of our cells depends on the efficiency of each step leading from gene to protein.

Proteins are the primary components of all plant and animal cells. Besides water and bones, protein is the major building material of our living bodies. Proteins are responsible for an unbelievably wide range of activities, from walking to curing a cold.

It is the shape that determines its biological activity and every typical protein is made up from folded amino acids, arranged in linear chains called polypeptide chains; a chain of 100 amino acids that could have up to 10^{100} (this means the number ten followed by one hundred zeros) possible configurations.

Our essence is carried on three-dimensional shapes informed by an electrical charge carried on an intracellular chemical fluid medium. Something like fantastically ornate origami party decorations floating in a charged cellulose river.

Yet – the extraordinary mind-blowing thing is not the complexity of everything; it is the simplicity.

DNA is actually extremely stable; studies of 50,000-year-old fossils show the DNA structure to be still intact and viable. We know that of the 92 chemical elements that occur in nature, the same small selection of 16 forms the basis of all living matter. From the thousands of possible combinations, just 20 amino acids are singled out as the units of construction for all proteins. Most significant of all, these proteins are produced in the right place at the right time by an ordered sequence of events governed by a code carried on just four molecules, called nucleotide bases. Of the possible contortions each protein could perform, each consistently chooses just one.

However, this tells us nothing about where we store the bananas.

*

With such a simple recipe, how is it we get so much complexity? Cellular biologists, neuroscientists and immunologists say the most significant part of the recipe above has very little to do with its various ingredients, but more to do with its movement.

It is not the number of amino acids that determine their function, it is their shape. At the tiniest level, a protein generates motion, literally 'energy', as it changes shape. This is controlled by electromagnetic charges along the protein's chain, and this movement gets harnessed to do 'work'.

The magic of life is in the compounded exchange of thousands of inputs of 'energy' – and its organisation.

Research published in mainstream scientific journals can clearly show that – beyond chemical information – pulsed electromagnetic fields regulate virtually every cell function.

Individual humans have unique frequencies associated with all their cell membrane receptors and thoughts emit the same variety of frequencies that activate biological processes within the cell.

As a consequence of these findings, Bruce Lipton argues: 'They are relevant for they acknowledge that biological behaviour can be controlled by "invisible" energy forces, these include thought'. We now recognise all those hundreds of thousands of receptors on each of our 50 trillion or so cells respond to energy signals as well as molecular signals; and carbon and hydrogen in DNA contribute to the mastery

173

of thought, feelings and time. Beyond our physical blueprint, our DNA is our repository of thoughts, feelings, dreams, wishes and intentions.

DNA itself is not made of anything special; it can be subdivided into simpler atoms of carbon, hydrogen, oxygen and so on. In other words, on a material level you, me, and a tree, are made up of mostly carbon, hydrogen, oxygen, nitrogen and a few other elements in minute amounts. In billions of other combinations, hydrogen and carbon simply exist.

The essential difference between a tree and us is the energy and information content of our bodies, as with a television where the tube, wires, metal bolts and circuit boards produce a picture only when they are all put together in a certain order. In the end, all the parts are necessary for a telly to exist. Yet, without the idea of 'telly', there would be no reason for all the parts to be together.

So, on the level of every cell, we respond and inform both thought and matter. It is the movement that is the miracle. The information, the impulse passing ceaselessly and without end around, through and over every little cell – the energy – where the miracle is.

That's the banana store – what we think and feel, whether it is about bananas or anything else, is carried throughout the body and changes the configuration of our proteins, which in turn hold that information for our minds to draw on when needed.

Consciously or unconsciously.

Thought is more than connected to the body, it is merged with the body. That is why we blush physically when we feel embarrassed, we cry when we watch a soppy film and we can taste bananas just thinking about them.

*

Behavioural biologist Paul Martin states: 'Our dualist habit of contrasting mind and body, as though they are two fundamentally different entities, is deeply misleading.'

The brain used to be thought of as a well-behaved complicated sack of hormones and enzymes organised by cells firing a linear single neurotransmitter across a synapse.

'Right now, that's at best a special case,' says Dr Steve Henricksen, senior staff scientist at the Salk Institute in La Jolla, California. According to him, 'Things are incredibly complex in the brain; we used to think the brain was like a computer, now we think each cell is like a computer, a separate computer. And one single cell is a whole brain.'

It has transpired that a neuron doesn't just catch and pass a signal untouched across a synapse. That is only one of its choices. The idea of an impulse travelling across a synapse does not take into account the information passing back along that synapse simultaneously in the opposite direction.

Do you remember the drawing of the eye in school? A silhouette of a person connected by dotted lines converging on the pupil, crossing, and inverting the picture on the back of the eyeball. I remember that's when the bell always went and I would leave for a break and gossip with that picture firmly in my mind. It took me more than a summer holiday to realise that we do not go around with an image of the world in miniature and upside down inside our heads.

What we actually see is people the right way up, precisely as they are and, more significantly, right where they are standing.

Right there and in that moment.

Brain connections don't go one way and wait for a reply; they are going all directions at once – and instantaneously – with powerful effects all over your body.

In 1982, Soft Cell's *Tainted Love* stayed in the charts for 35 weeks and defined the summer. It was a long, hot, summer of New Romantic fashion, lots of make-up and a great need to build the tallest hair or have it cut in the strangest angles.

But at the University of Paris, a research team, led by physicist Alain Aspect, performed what may turn out to be one of the most important experiments of the twentieth century. His team discovered that sub-atomic particles such as electrons are able – regardless of distance – to instantaneously communicate with each other. It doesn't matter if they are ten feet or ten billion miles apart.

The neurons that compose the brain talk to each other across synapses, which are gaps that separate tiny branch-like filaments called dendrites, which grow at the ends of each nerve cell. Each of us possesses billions of these cells; each one is capable of growing dozens or even hundreds of dendrites.

Meaning that at any one time, the possible combination of signals jumping across the synapses of the brain exceeds the number of atoms in the known universe.

*

Apparently, more than 95 per cent of the population came into this world with an intact genome for a healthy and fit existence; so the interesting question is why the majority of us, who possess a fit genome, acquire dysfunction and disease.

To say the mind and body are one is not to imply that disease is the product of 'incorrect' or 'negative' thinking, which is not only unhelpful, it is an abominably poor version of the truth. It is more helpful to accept the mind and body are one and go from there.

The 'placebo effect' does more than indicate that material, environmental, and mechanical exchanges are inadequate explanations of all that influence our health.

Our brains can make any reaction happen and then, more importantly, take it all away again, just as neatly as it began.

The Greek philosopher Epicurus (341 BC) argued two thousand years ago that the mind is one of the flexible forces that influence the body's health and its response to disease.

- Of the ninety two that occur in nature, the same selection of 16 chemical elements form the basis of all living matter.

- From the thousands of possible combinations, just 22 amino acids are singled out as the units of construction for all protein.

- Most significant of all, these proteins are produced in the right place at the right time by a code carried on just four nucleotide bases.

- Of the possible contortions every protein could perform each consistently chooses just one.

With doctorates in anthropology and ethology and degrees in botany, chemistry, geology, geography, marine biology, and ecology, Dr of Philosophy and author Lyall Watson speaks nine languages and has worked as a palaeontologist. As he puts it 'This is true whether the protein is destined to become a bacterium or a Bactrian camel. The instructions for all life are written in the same simple language.'

16. Mind Depends on Matter

Psychoneuroimmunological studies have overwhelmingly demonstrated that mind, immunity and health are interrelated. From the laboratory to field studies, they have shown that psychological factors have an effect on the immune system, which in turn affects physical health and so the opposite is true too. We should accept that we can work not only with the body, it would be smart to work with the mind too. There are several ways we can do this:

- Self-disclosure, or 'talk therapies' cannot only improve how we feel, but make our lymphocytes more responsive and produce better immune function too. Self-disclosure often helps us formulate solutions to problems too.

- Guided imagery, visualisation and active trance-therapies, or hypnotic relaxation techniques have been shown to aid diagnosis and promote physiological function and indeed boost the T-lymphocyte levels in blood.

- Behavioural therapies like CAT (Cognitive Analytic Theory) and belief therapies (using such techniques as Neurolinguistic Programming (NLP) like 'The Journey', especially those designed to facilitate the emotions of hopelessness, helplessness or worthlessness, have proved empirically successful.

- Relaxation therapy has proved to work with medical problems as diverse as hypertension and recurrent mouth ulcers to alopecia (hair loss) with changes in T-lymphocyte levels and beta-endorphin levels. A hobby can have the same effect.

- Self-healing traditions like Qi Gong promote health, fitness and longevity. Group therapy, music, art or dance maintain and improve both mental and physical health.

Thought, emotions and consciousness have growing explanations as physical processes, as Aristotle put it 'like sight is to the eye'. As such, they have a valid place to be considered in any question of health and treatment.

Both matter and mind matter.

17. A Smile Can Buy You Immunity

❝ A portrait painted on a panel is at once a picture and a likeness: that is, while one and the same, it is both of these, although the "being" of both is not the same, and one may contemplate it either as a picture, or as a likeness. ❞

Sigmund Freud

*

Have you ever noticed that the moment that your child unlocks a laugh from deep down inside you is absolutely the same moment that you feel better than you have ever felt before?

It turns out there is a good reason for this.

Arguably one of the sweetest things I have ever learnt is that an immune cell is not only able to defend you against a pathogen, but it is also capable of feeling happy. More importantly, feeling happy and being well are – to the immune system – the same thing. A good giggle is the peak of health.

Happy people don't get colds.

Psychopharmacological findings show that when that happy feeling is flowing through us it binds to the exact same antennae on a cell as those used by the cold virus. If all the antennae have an occupied sign put up by feeling happy there is no vacancy for the virus.

When we are happy we are, in that instant, exuberantly healthy. Neuroscientists have found they can link a more healthy response to immunisation shots with positive temperaments. It is not a coincidence that research shows happy people have more activity in their left prefrontal cortex, are more psychologically resilient, open to experiences, assertive, and empathetic. They are also much less likely to fall ill and live longer than unhappy people.

Some argue that health cannot be defined as a state at all, but should be seen as a process of continuous adjustment to the changing demands of living and of the changing meanings we give to our life events. How we feel shapes how healthy we can be.

To the immune system, the difference between health and stress is as subtle as our attitude to clutter.

You know that feeling when you walk into a room at the end of a day and all you can see is the mess: the toys on the floor, the puddle of spilt juice, the biscuit crumbs. The last thing you want to do is deal with this 'natural disaster' and you immediately feel worn out.

Or – I am told – you can feel entirely different. Apparently natural disasters occur only when hazards meet vulnerability and, if the mess does not bother you it is like an earthquake happening in an empty desert.

You can – so I am told – enter the disaster area (sitting room) and see only the space you love being in and think 'and it would look so much better if I just scooped up these few things cluttered about'.

These two approaches are roughly the choices our immune cells have to respond to life. The body changes physiologically to a threat to our health, either as a huge clean-up operation or as nothing but a bit of debris to be cleared, while it gets on with the important thing of being healthy.

Which, by default, also means happy.

The significance of this is that our immune systems themselves make that choice, and can manufacture substances for either defence or happiness.

Not only are our mind and body linked, but our body is capable of thinking for itself – and, in fact, does a lot of our thinking for us.

At the dawn of history, in the world of the protozoa, each cell was innately intelligent, an independent being adjusting its biology to its own perception of the environment.

As the world of cells got more complicated they joined to form multicellular 'communities'. The cells of a multicellular organism – of which we are an example – cannot behave independently; to survive they must cooperate. Contrary to popular belief, survival depends on co-operation, not competition. For us, don't forget, that is a community of around 70 trillion single cells.

However, as well as being an upstanding member of the community, each cell is a sophisticated individual too. One that can 'read' its environment, assess the information and then select appropriate behavioural programmes to maintain its survival.

Work done by the cellular biologist at Stanford University in the US, Bruce Lipton, actually shows that a cell thinks for itself; its 'brain' is its membrane. Our cell membrane is interacting with its environment, and with us inside, how we feel about things. With everything we go through, including our thoughts, actions and emotions.

A cell is also capable of having emotions of its own and signalling them to our brains.

At a cellular level, these minute physiological phenomena, in all parts of the body and brain, can – and do

– translate into large, full-body changes in activity, behaviour and even mood.

This tiny, choreographed spectacle of reciprocal interactions between receptors and 'informational substances' goes on simultaneously in different directions, dozens, hundreds, thousands of times, over a network of 70 billion or so cells. While regulating motor control and maintaining body functions, cells are processing sensation, thoughts and emotions too.

But every cell also informs thought.

This is true for each cell of our immune system; they too have their say in what they feel and do.

*

The work neuroscientists are doing with neuropeptides shows this two-way relationship, and the story began with the opiate receptor. On 25 October 1972, while Don Mclean was singing bye bye to 'American Pie', and *The Godfather* played the screens, a young graduate PhD student, Candace B. Pert, discovered the opiate receptor (one molecule on the surface of a cell). This led to the identification of the endorphin.

This was a breakthrough moment.

Unless our body has a receptor for a substance it will consider it a foreign substance. So, when Ms Pert set to thinking about opium she realised that the human body could only respond to the drug if we already had a receptor to take delivery of a substance like opium. If there was already a receptor, it meant we had to be naturally producing a very similar drug to opium within ourselves.

Hence the discovery of endorphins, a group of ten internally-produced morphine-like substances responsible for an array of drug-like effects in the body. Scientists believed endorphins would explain everything from falling asleep to falling in love.

But the endorphin rush didn't last long; it got complicated.

Now, endorphin was/is only one of the substances altering our moods at the cellular level. So the idea of the 'endorphin' was not enough to cover the many internal chemicals that were identified month by month in laboratories across the world. They began to defy classification, so somebody changed the name to neuropeptides.

But they work the same way despite the re-branding: every neuropeptide is a molecular messenger, designed to bind with a particular type of receptor on cells and deliver the specific information they need.

For example, a 'happy' neuropeptide will only bind with a happy receptor, and so on for moods like excitement, embarrassment, love and so forth.

At the same time, the immunologists were discovering that the immune system made informational substances too, and called them cytokines and chemokines.

But, the research findings were confusing, and then contradictory.

Eventually, people figured out that everyone was looking at the same molecules. There is an African saying: 'A lion and a buffalo should not fight to decide which of them is a snake.'

Scientists finally grasped the fact that the endorphins, or happy molecules, are made everywhere in our bodies, including our immune system.

Dr Candace B. Pert, in her seminal work *Molecules of Emotion,* remarks: 'Endorphin receptors, while densely concentrated in the limbic brain, also occur in every other part of our body.' The implication is that an emotion – like happiness – occurs in the blood, organs, muscles, tissue, and bone at the same time as it registers in the limbic system of our brain.

So emotions like 'happy' not only happen in our brains but also happen in our bodies. First we feel it, then the message passes through the limbic system and then it is sent to the frontal cortex – and only at this point do we finally know – consciously notice – we are feeling 'happy'.

*

The discovery of neuropeptides was so significant because it showed that cells all over the body were manufacturing these substances independent of the brain. It was realised that our immune system is capable of making 'informational substances' for itself; it behaves like a brain.

As we know, the brain makes immune-modulating chemicals called interleukins; at a physical, practical level these are 'coaches' that help the immune system adapt to circumstances. However, immune cells themselves are also known to make interleukins. For example, T-helper cells in a brawl with an infection produce interleukin 2 which tells other infection-fighting cells to multiply and mature.

In addition, our immune system cells can also make, store and secrete neuropeptides – the emotion potions – the same chemicals that we regard as controlling our moods.

Interleukins and neuropeptides are essentially the same, the difference in function is very small.

- Interleukins are produced to sort out things that happen to us, from cuts and bruises to infections.

- Neuropeptides are produced to sort out how we feel about what happens to us.

However, at a molecular level, there is so little difference between interleukins and neuropeptides; it is as slight as an inflection on the end of the word 'yes'. The word 'yes' is the same in every way except that with an inflection it is a question, and without an inflection 'yes' is an answer.

Both interleukins and neuropeptides are of the immune system as well as the brain.

Just as physical trauma causes the release of the body's defence mechanisms, so *feeling* wounded can cause the brain to release the peptide norepineprine, which has a similar effect on the body as histamine.

This communication between nervous and immune systems is a network of simultaneous messages and responses, with both physical and emotional triggers.

However, ground-breaking work on neuropeptides in the early 1980s showed immune cells seem to go beyond just fighting the good cause; they are also capable of being happy.

More significantly, being happy is as effective a defence against disease as being on the attack can be. Perhaps more so.

Viruses use the same receptors on our cells as neuropeptides do and, according to psychoneuro-immunologist Dr Candace B. Pert, 'depending on how much of the natural peptide for a particular receptor is around and available, the virus that fits that receptor will have an easier or harder time getting into a cell'. She goes on to explain that the rheovirus (the one which has been shown to be the cause of viral colds) uses the same receptor to enter a cell as the one for 'happy'. When you are happy, the rheovirus – cold – can't enter your cells because your happy feeling is taking up all the receptors that a virus could potentially use.

Our minds and bodies have two choices about how they respond to our environment and experiences: they can protect us or they can grow. We can moan about the clutter or we can just sweep it away while concentrating on all the good things.

Both are a way to be healthy.

One means our bodies are in the fight or flight mode. This is obviously useful and sometimes necessary, but involves over-secretion of the immune-suppressing chemicals, like adrenalin and cortisol. Blood is shut off to the forebrain and diverted to the limbic system and lingering in the 'protection mode' can in due course destroy the body's defences, not least because normal replacement of protein – the main working parts of all cells – cannot happen.

Experimental evidence also shows the body does the same when we experience grief, feelings of failure, suppression of anger, and other 'negative' emotions. Besides physical bracing, prolonged stress can also result in 'psychological bracing', so we even begin to form beliefs and values that we use to protect ourselves.

You know: all those thoughts that begin with 'can't'.

The other way means our bodies (and minds) are taking things in their stride; we prevent disease and dysfunction, normal maintenance of homeostasis is carried out easily and we are happy – which is the same as healthy.

Investigations into laughter have found that what happens inside our body is the reverse of the stress response; levels of adrenalin and cortisol drop significantly.

Our immune system can make happy chemicals, which keep us well, and being well is the body's equivalent of being happy.

Maybe that's why we are always searching for happiness; because we never feel better than when we are happy.

The whole body is a thinking, creative expression of intelligence.

This includes the immune system.

Capable of thinking and feeling for itself, the immune system can be either in protection or growth; and growth is a very effective defence, arguably the most effective.

*

18. Just Before I Go

'Drugs are not always necessary. Belief in recovery always is.'

Norman Cousins, Adjunct Professor of Medical Humanities for the School of Medicine, University of California

*

There were cats, two of them, long-haired silky ones. And carpets, three inch thick pile ones. We had travelled a couple of hours to stay the weekend with friends, the ones with the cats. We wanted to see them, they had moved house, had a new baby and it was a big number birthday. It was meant to be 48 hours of fun. Unfortunately, Ben was allergic to their cats, and he was having a rough time.

We had to resort to using his volumatic spacer, his 'nose bottle'. He spent those two days clutching it like Dumbo with a feather. He relied on it to help him breathe.

This is not what you want for your child.

You never want to contemplate your child unable to breathe without help, you never want to go back to the steroids and you never want to see that nose-bottle 'thing' as a regular accessory ever again.

It just doesn't go with anything, in the way a nice handbag does.

Ben had been so well for so long it was a shock to have him ill and to need conventional medicine. Watching him, holding him, reassuring him, helping him however I could, all I could think about was the three weeks we were about to spend with my family. They had two cats, double-coated, drooly old moggies. How was I going to get this kid through that experience?

The allergy-causing material from cats isn't cat hair, but more accurately a protein present in the dander and saliva of cats. These cat allergens become airborne in the immediate environment as microscopic particles which, when inhaled into the nose or lungs, can trigger the immune system to attack.

The symptoms are produced by our body's immune functions working to neutralise a perceived threat. It is these functional reactions that conventional medicine is so good at stopping; however, I really thought we could do without lurching into crisis; we should be able to live day-to-day without needing emergency intervention.

How could a kid that's actually well, be so ill?

Allergies are a perfect demonstration of how our body and its immune system are linked to our environment and our emotions and to our mind. Allergies are a functional issue; there is something in the environment that is the 'cause', but our reaction – the 'effect' – is because of the 'meaning' for us. Ben's immune system has learned to give a certain 'meaning' to cat dander, for example.

In normal processing, cat dander, dust, pollen, etc., are innocuous substances; in the allergic response there is no germ, bacteria, virus or parasite involved. Our immune system turns into an overprotective mother who won't let friends over to play.

The cells that would typically take care of anything that you breathe in, like hay, grass, dust, etc., are those scavengers macrophages. They actually look like a little squid with long tentacles for suckering onto any alien that may get into your body. Our macrophages roam around foraging and eating benign foreign substances (like cat dander) all the time in the low level – 'the passive immune system' – response.

However, they are also responsible for the carnage; when a macrophage happens upon a virus, it munches away but signals frantically 'stranger danger' to alert the rest of the immune system. Helper T-cells rush to the scene to confirm things and our single-minded Killer T-cells arrive and explode the enemy (by injecting it with a chemical like histamine) without stopping to ask questions.

The immune system is an infinitely perceptive and responsive organic network. It can learn from just one contact with anything, from a cold to tuberculosis, to recognise it again. It retains information about each subtle contact and recalls the appropriate response instantly, almost out of habit.

'Appropriate' is the key word here.

A virus is a simple creature that procreates by taking over your cells to do it, which means your cells are raped and pillaged for the benefit of what is essentially a parasite. Nobody wants that, no, we want our Killer T-cells in there detonating the little virus, and the collateral damage to our own infected cells is acceptable if it means the defeat of the enemy.

But an allergy is no virus.

And healthy cells are being destroyed for no good reason.

It is an inappropriate response to perceive cat dander, pollen, grasses, dust and mites, etc., as dangerous.

For some reason, the body has learnt and memorised an inappropriate reaction, unleashing the 'active immune system' response. Because our systems are so darn clever (even when they are wrong) every time they recognise the same, or similar, substances they unleash their full might.

Ben's system had exhaustively learnt to recognise and confront the smallest amount of cat dander. Apart from being a pain in the chest, throat, nose, eyes and ears and all over inconvenient, if not downright debilitating, it is unnecessary – he was not under threat. He was not 'growing', because he was protecting himself against shadows and phantoms. He had to go through all the drag of feeling ill when he should have been having a good time.

Disease, allergies and immunisation teach us that the amazing wonder of our immune system is its ability to learn.

And if your immune system can think and learn, then is it possible that it can relearn patterns of immune response?

*

This all sounds like we sit around waiting for things to go wrong, when the opposite is true. In 1995, a new subset of T-cells was isolated; these appear to function exclusively as a brake on the immune system. Named regulatory T-cells, their role is to secrete chemicals that stop other Helper T-cells in their tracks. Experiments have shown that instead of our immune systems doing nothing until provoked, in fact they have to be held back. They are on the hunt all the time and have to be taught 'self-control'.

As good as we are at rapid response, we actually have to learn how to use the 'brakes'.

How often in this life is it true that the challenge is self-discipline?

Since 1984, scientists in the field of Neurolinguistic Programming (NLP) have been looking at the 'learned response' area of health. Based on successful psychotherapies and communication systems, NLP is the science of how we think, and the language patterns we use to store experiences. Robert Dilts is a highly respected author, developer and consultant working in the field of NLP. He explains: 'Illness is a function of interactions in your biological and neurological systems. It is a systemic process that is not related solely to any one thing. Some illnesses involve very complex systemic interactions – others are simpler.'

He goes on to point out that, 'In fact, some physical problems, like many allergic responses, are stimulus-response phenomena and can be changed using very quick and simple mental processes.'[33]

A human immune system that has an underdeveloped regulatory T-cell function can simply be too ready to launch an aggressive Helper T-cell response generating allergies; the immune system has no memory created of a 'self-possessed' response.

Suzi Smith is an NLP Master Practitioner with a special interest in health and assisting people to have more personal control over their wellbeing. She knows of children as young as three years old with allergies who have responded to NLP. She explains: 'Because your immune system learns so quickly, that means it is very teachable.' With allergies particularly they have proved you can teach your immune system an appropriate response. You can tell it that the response it is having now is unnecessary. We can say to our immune system, 'Not this response, *this* response.' Not this, *this*.

Suzi says, 'It's just a matter of retraining.'

The cells involved in active immune responses are produced in our bone marrow at the rate of about 80 million cells per minute, which can mean re-education can be rapidly effective.

*

Hypnosis has been shown in trials to speed the recovery of burns. Many studies have found that patients who believe a cure will work, whether it is a teaspoon of lemon juice or full conventional medical intervention, go on to recover in contradiction to prognosis. The placebo is a well-known phenomena of the power of the mind and body in health.

Dr Mosaraf Ali, the UK's leading pioneer of Integrated Medicine, director of the Integrated Health Centre in London, and best-selling author of several books, has been a practising conventional doctor and trained in seven other healing methods including acupuncture and Ayurveda over 20 years. He maintains that the body is capable of healing itself; it needs only the right conditions to be able to do so.

As a girl I remember all sorts of things – inexplicable 'miracles' going on around me. I particularly remember one day when Kabras, our head-milker on the farm, said to my father, 'Soita na Kwisha Kufa.' The three of us were standing looking at the horizon. The vast silences of Africa are an experience of the body, growing and permeating and rising until, when they are gone, it is as if a part of you is missing. You can end up searching restlessly for another moment you can enter that silence again.

'What can I do?' asked my father. Kabras shrugged. He had just told my father was that one of the farm hands had 'finished dying'.

He was the third worker in as many weeks to die of diagnosed TB, which had all the farm labourers whispering 'black magic'.

'And Wakesa?' my father asked.

Kabras shrugged again, as his mind disappeared off past the horizon for the answer. He then replied 'Shauri ya Mungu', an African saying meaning, it's in God's hands.

Just the week before, Wakesa had been taken to the doctor, consumed by the fever, wracked by a cough and bent over double under the strain of sitting in the back of a pick-up truck. It was a long, rutted, 12 miles to the doctor and my father helped to carry him to the fly-covered bench that served as a consulting table.

The missionary doctor examined him and diagnosed late-stage tuberculosis and assigned him a bed, wanting to get him on the drugs as soon as possible to have the best chance of saving him.

Wakesa had refused.

They explained to him what would happen if he did not accept help, and still he refused.

In Africa, your family accompanies you to the hospital to carry out your everyday care, and Wakesa had his brother with him. He too supported Wakesa's wish to leave the hospital. When they got back to the farm, my father explained he was going to let Wakesa go back to his tribal home.

Typically in Africa the men live where they can find work, often several hundred miles from their village. They go home only to father a child, and return to see the child for the first time on their first birthday.

My parents felt, as they waved goodbye to a man half his former self, it was the last time they would see him. He would be lucky to survive the three or four-day journey.

They were letting him return to his home to die.

Soon after that a man strode onto the farm with a gleaming white smile set in the shiny, healthy, deep chocolate colour of his face. Still a little thin, Wakesa was nevertheless ready to milk cows again.

We had the missionary doctor examine him and he could find no trace of TB anywhere. Shrugging his shoulders, the Doc said he had seen many a thing he could not explain. Wakesa's version was the witchdoctor in his village had removed a curse put on the entire farm.

Whatever the cause of the sickness, there never was another case of TB on the farm after that.

And it would seem Wakesa had recovered from an illness that, without treatment, he was predicted to die from. A little set intention, some bones banged on a bowl of herbs probably, a bit of belief, the support he received from his family and Wakesa's control of his own treatment had done the job, in contradiction to conventional wisdom.

Whatever it was, it worked; the right conditions were created for him to get better.

*

I read Suzi Smith's accounts of her case studies and the technique, called the Fast Allergy Process, and I was intrigued; it was non-invasive, non-addictive and, if it didn't have the desired outcome, it caused no harm. It followed all the rules and was a way to teach the immune system to put on the brakes: to re-learn an inappropriate response.

I was pretty sure I wanted Ben to see her as soon as possible. I told him we were going to try to get him some help with his allergies. I explained that it was something a little different; it could even be fun if he was willing to give it a try.

Of course he wanted to know what it involved.

We were walking down the street to our house at the time and I stepped in pace with him; we were both lazily wandering along, speaking in an easy-going manner.

I explained to him how smart his immune system was; how it could heal a cut, make a bruise better and fight colds – all without him having to think about it. How it had fought off the chickenpox without anybody else having to do anything. I explained the mistake his immune system had made with allergies and this meant it could learn not to do it any more, quickly and easily.

I then asked him if he liked having allergies for any reason at all. Was there anything good about them? He was pretty sure they were an 'all-round horrible thing to suffer'.

Then I recall I stopped and he turned to me and I brushed his hair behind his ears, held his hand and asked him if there was anything like cats he could think of that he wasn't allergic to.

He immediately answered: 'Dogs.'

We agreed they were like cats; they had fur and four legs and were pets that you could cuddle and they love you back.

'Mummy,' Ben said, 'that's how I want to feel with cats. I want to be able to get you another cat so there is a girl in the house for you.'

I hugged him, as I reassured him I loved my boys and they were enough and I wanted him to be able to have any pet he wanted and not to have to worry about allergies.

We carried on walking hand in hand and I asked him how it would feel if he could have a cat. We chatted about that and tried to imagine all the pets we could have and what it would be like, and soon we were outside the front door. I let him have the key to open the door for us and said he could think about it and to let me know if he wanted to try out this technique we had just talked about.

Two days later we were walking down the street again and Ben just came out with a very surprised: 'Mummy, it's gone!'

I was a bit distracted. 'What's gone, Benjamin bunny?'

'I used to have a sign here.' And he pointed to a space somewhere in front of his face. 'A sign, just here, of a red circle with a red line through the middle and a black silhouette of a cat behind it.'

He was waving his hand in front of and above his right eye, and telling me a picture had gone from his mind.

A week later we were sitting on a sofa covered in cat hairs, stroking a moulting cat, which was pushing up against Ben's face and purring.

He was having no reaction. Well, no negative one. He was actually a very happy little boy to be able to cuddle a cat and be loved back.

On the stroll home that day, Ben had, in effect, reprogrammed his immune system response and he no longer showed any signs of having an allergic reaction. In that brief chat, he had pulled off what seems impossible, but has been repeated hundreds of times in many countries. He and his immune system were smart enough to do it without even thinking about it.

Things that seem miraculous have a perfectly natural explanation. If they seem extraordinary it is only because we aren't familiar with the cause – yet.

At the first belief and health seminar Robert Dilts conducted, a researcher in the field of immunology and genetics was a guest speaker. The winner of the World Health Association Award for his definitive work in the 1950s, demonstrating that viruses are infectious, Dr Michael Levi commented that an allergy was like a phobia of the immune system. This resonated with other observations Dilts had made and, working initially with a biofeedback device that measures subtle physical changes, he discovered the types of brain processes involved with allergies. He developed an allergy retraining process, which Suzi Smith and her colleague Tim Hallbom, through experimentation, refined into a Fast Allergy Process.

The conversation between Ben and I had casually followed this procedure. I was intending only to explain it, not aiming to enact it; he knew nothing about it.

Ben still seldom shows a reaction to cats to this day.

*

- Calibrate. Ask, 'What's it like for you when you're in the presence of the allergen?' Watch the person's physiology, how they breathe, look, feel, etc. They will usually display allergic symptoms.

- Explain the mistake their immune system has made. It has marked out something as dangerous that's not, but it can learn so easily it can be retrained quickly.

- Check for secondary gains. What would life be like without this? Are there any positive or negative consequences? The purpose of identifying such positive intentions and secondary gains is to help the person add more choices. An underlying principal of NLP is that ecological change comes by adding new choices, not by taking away existing choices.

- Find an appropriate counter-example resource. Find something similar to the allergen that the immune system responds to appropriately; suggestive of the like-for-like principle and the way immunisation works. Then *anchor* (touch) the person and hold that touch throughout the process.

- Have the person dissociate. See themselves somewhere else, maybe behind a glass wall responding well to the allergen. Suggest to them that that is the person they want to be and that their immune system operates appropriately.

- *Gradually* introduce the allergen into that picture. Introduce it slowly enough for the person to get used to it. At this point, there should be a physiological 'shift', like the immune system saying, 'I get it, I will change that.'

- Reassociate. Bring them back into their body and have them imagine themselves in the presence of the allergen while you continue to hold your touch on them.

◆ Future pace. Have them imagine a time in the future when they will be in the presence of the thing that used to create an allergic response for them.

◆ Test. Carefully test them if you can. If you can't, re-calibrate to see if their physiology – breathing, look, feeling – has changed. They should show no allergic symptoms.

In working with allergies, as with any medical problem, it's important to do so in conjunction with appropriate medical treatment and/or professional help. Before you try these techniques be sure the person you are working with is under the supervision, or the treatment of, a qualified medical practitioner. Or seek the help of a trained professional with appropriate experience.

(Reprinted here with kind permission from: Robert Dilts, Suzi Smith and Tim Hallbom.)

The 4th Rule

Do most good

19. Do Most Good

I am always asking the boys how it is, after being pregnant for nine months each, giving very painful births, and being left with stretch marks like storylines across my stomach, that I still love them?

Considering I have changed their nappies for a combined ten and a half years and didn't sleep for nine years, we are in general agreement that, based on the evidence, I must love them a lot.

The truth, of course is, that whatever it takes, we want the best for our children, to do the best by them.

The last – and usually considered the most important – of Hippocrates' directives is to 'do least harm'.

Throughout this journey that I and Ben, and his brother Harry, have gone through, The 4th Rule has grown more relevant. I would argue it is the most significant. It is not the most significant just because some bloke, from an ancient time, believed it to be his best idea. It is his most important idea because it encapsulates our understanding of the best healthcare. It has proved itself over a very long time, across the planet.

Hippocrates' actual words were 'As to diseases make a habit of two things – to help, or at least, to do least harm.'

As a mum, I would say we don't just want to 'do least harm'.

We want to 'do most good'.

When I was first faced with Ben's prognosis, I felt conflicted, between accepting he only had allergies and asthma, and wanting the world to be perfect for my child. There were so many worse things that could be wrong with him and he was going to be relatively OK, but one time in A&E is one more than you want – no matter why you are there.

Knowing what we know now, I truly believe that had we completed the immunisation course as usual at Ben's fourth and fifth months of life, we would be placing pointless posies of flowers on a headstone every third Sunday of the month. Had I accepted there was nothing to do but manage his condition, we would probably have had to live with severe allergies, eczema, asthma, intermittent ear surgery and steroids, with all the side-effects and learning difficulties, for a further decade or more.

It took me a while to realise that he couldn't be 'fixed' by doctors, specialists, medicine, treatments or procedures.

Or me.

I learnt this as I became more aware of the truth that only he could fix himself.

All that I could do was help provide the right conditions for him to do so.

I could only do that if I knew where to start.

To stop and think what is the least harmful path to go down focuses your thoughts. Is it more harmful to allow the child to struggle with breathing – for a long time – with the resulting unknown and long-term physical and psychological effects? Or, is it more harmful to administer steroids – that work immediately – with the known and well-documented, long-term, side effects this has on the child's physiology?

It may take a moment or two to think it through. You have to ask; why are you in this situation, what are the immediate circumstances, and what is coming up over the next few days? And you also have to ask yourself when you are going to have time to do more than do the least harm?

Then the right question is: what will 'do most good'?

Are you doing what's best for you child?

When deciding a treatment, this is the most valuable guideline; it brings in a whole care package of possibilities. Dr Mosaraf Ali points out that, since healthcare was first recorded, practitioners have noticed: 'Health is governed by natural laws and to restore it you have to simply create a suitable environment for the body's natural ability to heal itself.'

Hippocrates himself said: 'The body heals itself, you need only to lay down the conditions.'

Because we, as mums, are experts in our own children, we know if there is 'something wrong'. It takes very little more to become better informed and take an active part in any decision about their health. Busy mums like us have a lot on our plates, but when I have been asked which single thing made the difference, the answer is that it wasn't any particular treatment or drug. It was that, as his mum I was the right person, in the right place, to make the right decision – and it is as simple as that.

The German pioneer of spinal anaesthesia (so useful in some labours), August Bier said: 'A smart mother often makes a better diagnosis than a poor doctor.' Knowing my child best, I could recognise what was valuable to him and I was there to see when things weren't working. Taking control of the health of your family requires that you view all treatments, procedures and medicines as both potentially helpful and potentially dangerous.

Ben, his body, did the hard work.

That is why this book is deliberately non-prescriptive; learning what questions to ask and how to judge the answers is so much more useful than simple instruction.

Asking questions, especially of doctors, is not something to be embarrassed about. You have the ability to understand any proposed course of action; you can learn what a doctor knows. Once upon a time he didn't know anything, either.

It is worth remembering that 50 per cent of all doctors graduate in the bottom half of their class.

This is true of any health practitioner, whatever their field.

You wouldn't expect to leave your kids at school without knowing anything about the school, because you just accepted it on face value, or you didn't want to be rude.

Tried and tested drugs don't work on everyone so while you may see the height of one man, it is not enough to give you the height of the human race. As J.H. Gaddum of London's National Institute for Medical Research, said: 'Patients may recover in spite of drugs, or because of them.'

After six years of research, across three continents, it became clear that there is no formula, 12-step plan, or cure-all, for all people. Modern medicine is exceptional at emergency care and surgery. Chronic conditions need an approach that creates the right conditions, as soil does for seeds, to allow the body to heal itself. The human body is suspended in a balanced fluid that is always responding to demands both physical and mental. The human body is complex and the solution can be, too, and that is why an integrated approach is often most successful. Understanding how our immune system works is really useful. However, I learnt the most important thing was the relationship between our bodies and the world of germs. I don't mean knowing all the Igs from A to E of the immune system, but just understanding survival of the fittest is a natural law.

Pioneer epidemiologist and director of the first municipal health laboratory in the US, Charles V. Chapin, said: 'It takes two to make a disease, the microbe and its host.'

I found it really helpful to understand that having a disease is very different to all the aches and pains and problems that are not caused by bugs. These symptoms are the result of dysfunction – when demands outstrip our resources.

This distinction is vital in order to make sense of a mosaic of symptoms and to make better decisions about how we treat ourselves. In context, we can understand that sometimes the situation demands that we stop things in their tracks, and sometimes we need to support our system to do what it knows best. The distinction helps us chose the appropriate drugs, treatments or procedures – or if a bit of rest, a better diet, or doing nothing is the best way to proceed.

Our physical forms are the result of 400 millions years of survival. They are highly complex and sophisticated. They are built and honed through direct experience of the planet with which we co-exist. They have developed beyond our understanding to withstand, and process, a great deal of battering. The brain, for example, produces narcotics up to 200 times stronger than anything you can buy on the high street, and our own pain-killers are non-addictive. When we attempt to replicate this with man-made drugs, the so-called active ingredient has no active 'intelligence'.

Even though the chemical make-up of adrenalin is identical, no matter where it is derived from, when it is injected into someone, the results are nowhere near as precise as our own adrenalin. Nor can they be modified and brought to an end. The drug floods the receptor sites on our cells and cannot recalled or neutralised.

From about the time of Hippocrates, the philosophy of health has been to gain an understanding of the natural order of things in order to grow in harmony with it.

Our best shot at prolonged health and happiness is to realise that our immune systems are vital to our endurance; they allow all the other systems of our body to function at their best.

We can do our best by our immune systems, and those of our children, if we start to learn what we are really looking at, and use this big picture to make decisions.

We mums are in a good position to do that because, as Hippocrates said: 'It is more important to know what sort of person has a disease than to know what sort of disease a person has.'

If we remember our kids are the unique creatures we know them to be and treat them as these individuals, we have a shot at doing better for them.

There are many ways in which we can prevent bad things happening to them, but the most effective way to equip them well for life is to prepare them so well that they seldom need help.

But, finally, the overriding guideline is to 'do least harm', or as most mums feel is more naturally right to 'do most good'.

The right question is always: what will do the most good?

How do we do this?

Remember there are two ways we can be ill; with a disease or dysfunction. There are two ways to treat conditions 'contrary to suffering' or 'like-for-like'.

And there are four rules:

- be guided by observations;
- treat people not disease;
- prevention is better than cure;
- do most good.

As Galen said: 'Confidence and hope do more good than physic.'

I do know, as a mum, that we make the best job of it for our kids, and that counts for a lot. If we were only able to choose one wish for our kids, I am sure most of us would say we want them to be happy. A healthy body and a happy outlook are – on a biological level – the same thing.

Health is not a physical state, it is an attitude.

Diseases wreck creation, but health is more about recreation.

We could spend less time discovering the causes of our problems and give more attention to the causes of health.

My children now eat their way through a weekly shop in two days, in fact Ben loves food enough he regularly cooks pasta meals for the family (thanks to Jamie Oliver). Homework gets done, social engagements are crammed into the spare hours. They are smart, handsome and funny, and yes I am their mum, but I have been able to stop worrying, and start enjoying too. What more could we want for our children?

And our families deserve it.

*

Go to bed between 10 and 11pm

Do some movement in the morning

Eat your biggest meal in the middle of the day

Spend time outside every day

Take in eight glasses of water a day

Meditate

Avoid drugs, legal or otherwise

Take responsibility for your own health decisions

Eat those fruit and veg

Do something really enjoyable, everyday

Apparently these are the top ten health habits that make the most difference. It is all normal stuff: it's a good time to go to bed, stretching eases the stiffness. It's easier to sleep on a light meal. There are skies even over cities. There is water in fruit and veg, so that makes it 2-for-1 and nobody needs an excuse for having a laugh. It is normal, real stuff that doesn't need fancy science or focusing on, so it shouldn't be that hard to fit all this into daily life.

Reference and Citation List

Every attempt has been made to seek permission for all references in the book and to cite work accurately, where it is quoted.

1. Gerd Gigerenzer, *Reckoning with Risk* (Penguin, 2002), p21.
2. *British Medical Journal*, 324: pp859–60, 13 April 2002.
3. Dr Phil Hammond and Michael Mosley, *Trust Me, (I'm a Doctor): A Consumer's Guide to How The System Works* (Metro, 1999), p96.
4. BBC Online allergy guide, 3 April 2002.
5. *Holistic Health*, no 73, summer 2002.
6. *British Medical Journal*, 324: pp859–60, 13 April 2002.
7. Extracted from Dr Andrew Weil's *Spontaneous Healing How to Discover and Embrace Your Body's Natural Ability to Maintain and Heal Itself* (Random House Publishing Group, New York).
8. R.M. Rosenfeld, J.E. Vertrees, J. Carr *et al.*, 'Clinical efficacy of antimicrobial drugs for acute otitis media: meta-analysis of 5400 children from thirty-three randomised trials', *Journal of Pediatrics*, 1994, 124: pp355–67.
9. Antibiotics for Acute Otitis Media, June 1995, 16–3, Bandoman Bandolier, Bandolier Library, search antibiotics for acute otitis media ear infections in children.
10. *New Scientist*, 8 June 2002, p5.
11. Lynne McTaggart, *What Doctor's Don't Tell You* (Thorsons), p186.

12. *The Guardian*, G2 section, 24 April 2003, p2.

13. Michael Hardt and Antonio Negri, *Empire* (Harvard University Press), p306.

14. Moynihan R., Heath I., Henry D., 'Selling Sickness: the pharmaceutical industry and disease mongering', *British Medical Journal*, 2002, 324: pp886–90.

15. Pbs.org/wgbh/aso/databank/entries/dm28pe.html

16. William Crook, *Solving the Puzzle of Your Hard-to-Raise Child* (Random House, New York, 1981).

17. Catherine J.M. Diodati, Immunization: History, Ethics Law, and Health, Windsor, Ontario: Integral aspects, 1999, p71.

18. Ricki Lewis, Paper for the US Food and Drug Administration, 'The Rise of Antibiotic-Resistant Infections'.

19. Department of Health, *Saving Lives: Our Healthier Nation* (DoH, 1999).

20. Dr Keith Scott-Mumby, *Virtual Medicine* (Thorsons, 1999), p4.

21. *The Integrated Health Bible*, Dr Mosaraf Ali, (Vermillion), p15.

22. The wave-like phenomena of visible light was a concept first proposed in the late 1600s by Dutch physicist Christian Huygens. Electromagnetic radiation is the main way energy travels through the universe.

23. a and b – Vol. 2 of the third edition of *The Letters and Works of Lady Mary Worley Montagu*, W.Moy Thomas (Henry G. Bohn, London, 1861), p308.

24. Geoff Watts, *Pleasing the Patients* (Wiley and Sons, 1982), p42.

25. T.D. Barnes, *Tertullian – A Historical and Literary Study* (Oxford: Clarendon Press, 1971).

26. Tertullian became a Christian but many writers (inc. Bardenhewer and Quasten) believe the *Apologeticum* to be autobiographical.

27. Harris L. Coulter and Barbara Loe Fisher, *A Shot in the Dark* (Avery Publishing Group), p122.

28. Selected essays by Richard Dawkins, *The Devil's Chaplin* (Weidenfeld and Nicholson, 2005), p31.

29. a-l All italicised references are taken from Coulter and Fisher, ibid.

30. Medhist.ac.uk – living city (1800 Year reference).

31. Ivan Illich, 'Medical Nemesis – the expropriation of health' (Calder and Boyars, 1975).

32. Campaign Against Fraudulent Medical Research Newsletter, 1995, 2(3): 5–13, quoting statistics from the London Bills of Mortality 1760–1834 and Reports of the Registrar General 1838–96, as compiled in Alfred Wallace, *The Wonderful Century* (1898).

33. Robert Dilts, Tim Hallbom and Suzy Smith, *Beliefs: pathways to health and wellbeing* (Metamorphous Press, 1990), p171.

List of Useful Contacts

I have drawn up this list as a resource for responsible, personal decisions, it is not an endorsement of any particular body or any particular therapy. Some organisations can give conflicting recommendations, so it would be wise to consider a range of viewpoints and come to your own health decisions.

British Holistic Medical Association, Trust House, Royal Shrewsbury Hospital South, Shrewsbury, Shropshire SY3 8XF

British Association for Holistic Health, 179a Gloucester Place, London NW1 6DX

Holistic Health Foundation, 2 De La Hay Avenue, Plymouth, Devon PL3 4HH

Council for Complementary and Alternative Medicine, 206–8 Latimer Road, London W10 6RE

British Complementary Medicine Association, 39 Presbury Road, Cheltenham, Gloucester GL52 2PT

Alternative Health Information Bureau, 12 Upper Station, Radlett, Hertfordshire WD7 8BX

Research Council for Complementary Medicine, 60 Great Ormond Street, London WC1N 3JF

General Council and Register of Osteopaths, 56 London Street, Reading, Berkshire RG1 4SQ

The British Chiropractic Association, Equity House, 29 Whitley Street, Reading RG2 0EG

Craniosacral Association, Monomark House, 27 Old Gloucester Street, London WC1N 3XX

Ayurvedic Medical Association UK, The Hale Clinic, 7 Park
    Crescent, London W1N 3HE

British Association for Counselling, 1 Regents Place, Rugby,
    Warwickshire CV21 2PJ

International Institute of Reflexology UK, 15 Hartfield Close,
    Tonbridge, Kent TN10 4JP

British Acupuncture Council, Park House, 206–208 Latimer
    Road, London W1N 3HE

The Council for Nutrition Education and Therapy, 1 The
    Close, Halton, Aylesbury, Buckinghamshire HP22 5NJ

British Hypnotherapy Association, 67 Upper Berkeley Street,
    London W1H 7DH

British Register of Complementary Practitioners, PO Box
    194, London SE16 1QZ

One of the most reliable, best-researched and impartial
websites is What Doctors Don't Tell You www.wddty.com

Please note that this information was as accurate as we could
make it at the time of going to press. Addresses and other
aspects are subject to change, so please be understanding
when using this material for reference.

Recommended Reading

I have read many books, from very conventional ones to some that have been from the far reaches of human experience. Listed here are those I enjoyed or learnt from, the two are not mutually exclusive.

Dr Mosaraf Ali, *The Integrated Health Bible* (Vermillion, London).

Dr Keith Scott-Mumby, *The Allergy Handbook* (Thorsons, London).

Lynne McTaggart, *What Doctors Don't Tell You: The Truth About the Dangers of Modern Medicine* (Thorsons, London).

Candace B. Pert, *Molecules of Emotion: Why You Feel the Way You Feel* (Pocket Books, London).

Coulter and Fisher, *A Shot in the Dark* (Avery Publishing Group Inc.).

Robert Dilts, Tim Hallbom and Suzi Smith, *Beliefs, Pathways to Health and Well-being* (Metamophous Press, Oregon).

Norman Cousins, *Anatomy of an Illness* (Bantum, New York).

Bernie Siegal, *Love, Medicine and Miracles: Lessons Learned About Self Healing from a Surgeon's Experience with Exceptional Patients* (HarperCollins, New York).

Lyall Watson, *Supernature* (Coronet, Hodder UK).

Bruce Lipton, *The Biology of Belief: Unleashing the Power of Consciousness, matter and miracles.* (Mountain of love Productions/Elite Books).

Gerd Gigerenzer, *Reckoning with Risk* (Allen Lane, The Penguin Press).

Paul Martin, *The Sickening Mind: Brain, Behaviour, Immunity and Disease* (Flamingo).

Dr Andrew Lockie and Dr Nicola Geddes, *Homeopathy: The Principles and Practice of Treatment* (Dorling Kindersley, London).

Dr Robert Mendelsohn, *Confessions of a Medical Heretic* (Contemporary Books, US).

Fritjof Capra, *The Tao of Physics: An Exploration of the Parallels Between Modern Physics and Eastern Mysticism* (Bantum, New York).

Deepak Chopra, *Ageless Body, Timeless Mind: The Quantum Alternative to Growing Old* (Harmony, New York).

Deepak Chopra, *Quantum Healing: Exploring the Frontiers of Mind/Body Medicine* (Bantum, New York).

Richard Dawkins, *The Selfish Gene* (Oxford University Press, Oxford).

Andrew Weil, *Spontaneous Healing: How to Discover and Enhance Your Body's Natural Ability to Maintain and Heal Itself* (Random House Publishing Group).

Dr Phil Hammond and Michael Mosley, *Trust Me (I'm a Doctor): A Consumer's Guide to How the System Works* (Metro).

Joseph O'Connor and John Seymour, Foreword by Robert Dilts, Preface by John Grinder, *Introducing Neuro-Linguistic Programming: The New Psychology of Personal Excellence* (Mandala, London).

Chris Ward and Simon Eccles, *So You Want to be a Brain Surgeon?* (Oxford University Press, Oxford).

David Peters (ed.), *Understanding the Placebo Effect in Complementary Medicine: Theory, Practice and Research* (Churchill Livingstone, University of Westminster).

Masuru Emoto, *Messages From Water: The World's First Pictures of Frozen Water Crystals* (Hado Kyoikusha Co., Japan).

Ivan Illich, *Medical Nemesis* (Calder and Boyars).

Pitirim Alexandrovich Sorokin, *Basic Trends in Our Times* (Rowman & Littlefield Publishers, 1964).

Robert Merton, *Social Theory and Social Structure* (Free Press, 1957).

Water Works

Despite it being common knowledge that water is a chemical compound of two of the most universal elements, hydrogen and oxygen, H_2O, no scientist can tell you exactly how it works.

Water is of major importance to all living things; the cells in our bodies are full of water, about 60–65 per cent of the human body is water, the brain is composed of 70 per cent water, blood is 82 per cent water, and the lungs are nearly 90 per cent water.

Vital for the haulage of waste material from our bodies, it is central for the metabolisation and transportation in the bloodstream of the carbohydrates and proteins that our bodies use as food.

Surface tension plays a part in our body's ability to transport these elements all through ourselves. Liquid water is so intricately laced that it is almost a continuous structure as opposed to several molecules bonded together. This gives it both extraordinary strength and flexibility. The excellent ability of water to dissolve so many substances allows our cells to use valuable nutrients, minerals, and chemicals in biological processes.

Water is called the 'universal solvent', although hydrochloric acid, as one of the strongest acids known readily attacks common metals, water can dissolve more substances than any other liquid. This means that wherever water goes, either through the ground or through our bodies, it takes along valuable chemicals, minerals, and nutrients.

Biological reactions need to happen quickly with little use of energy and, because the links between its atoms are easily broken, water makes an ideal, universal, trigger substance. No scientist doubts that water behaves like this inside a plant, animal or indeed us.

Between 35 and 40 degrees centigrade, water is particularly unstable, and therefore most valuable to life, and this is the body temperature of most active animals.

Water has a high 'specific heat index', meaning water can absorb a lot of heat before it begins to get hot. That is why it is used in car radiators as a coolant. It is because of the water in the air that the changes between seasons are gradual.

Water's freezing and boiling points are the baseline with which temperature is measured: $0°$ on the Celsius scale is water's freezing point, and $100°$ is water's boiling point. Yet it responds to changes in air pressure; at the beach it will boil at $100°C$, but at 5,000 feet you will need less fuel for a cup of tea as it boils at $94.9°C$, and half way up a mountain like Kilimanjaro at 10,000 feet it boils at $89.8°C$. It is denser in the liquid state that in its solid forms. Heating it up from 0 to 4 degrees above melting point causes it to become most dense. Ice forms the most perfectly bonded hydrogen structure known. Its crystalline pattern is so precise we can tell, even though it looks regular to us, a glass of tap water contains short lived spots of ice crystals that form and melt many millions of times every second. It is even thought that ice-like areas form in hot water.

It can act as an acid and as a base, actually reacting chemically with itself under certain conditions. Neutral water (such as distilled water) has a pH of 7. Seawater happens to be slightly alkaline (basic), with a pH of about 8. Most natural water has a pH of between 6 and 8, and acid rain can have a pH as low as 4.

It has the tensile strength of many metals and there isn't a container strong enough to hold pure water.

It is unique in being the only natural substance that can exist in all three states of solid (ice), liquid (water), and gas (vapour) at the same time, at the temperatures normally found on Earth. Earth's water is continuously interacting, changing, and flowing from one to the other in a cycle, also known as the hydrologic cycle, in which there is no beginning or end. These processes can happen in the blink of an eye and over millions of years. Although the balance of water on Earth remains fairly constant over time, individual water molecules can come and go in a hurry. Created by an act of Congress in 1879, the US Geological Survey, the sole science agency for the Department of the Interior, has vast earth and biological data holdings. They have charted that the water in the apple you ate yesterday may have fallen as rain half-way around the world last year or it could have been bathed in by a plesiosaurus 100 million years ago.

In tests, water has shown an amazing ability to 'remember', to store information about what it comes into contact with, whether it is chemical, electromagnetic waves or mechanical pressures like sound.

A German test, by H. Teichman, found that a thimbleful of rose scent diluted in a lake covering fourteen thousand square miles can be recognised by eels sensitive to that body of water as distinct from all others as reported in *Naturewiss* 44: 242 in 1957.

Work with phenylthiocarbamide, or PTC, the most famous bitter flavour, has shown that some people can still taste it in the practically absent dilution of 18 parts per billion.

A Japanese researcher, Masaru Emoto, has photographed frozen water crystals under laboratory conditions. He has shown, many times, that water forms different crystals when exposed to different influences, it 'remembers'. He took 100 test tubes of distilled water and wrote the same word on the glass, the word 'love', and then he left them in a freezer for 24 hours. He took another 100 test tubes and wrote 'hate' on them and left them to freeze for 24 hours. Then he photographed the crystals formed under high magnification. The ones with 'love' on had all formed near perfect crystals. The ones with 'hate' on uniformly failed to form crystals.

In his book *Message from Water* he shows experiments with other words, music and pictures. He took distilled water and photographed it before using it when it barely forms misshapen crystals. He then left a sample of the water on a photograph of a happy child, when it then formed perfect crystals. He has also done some work with dilutions of substances. Milk diluted 200 times forms a distinct crystal, when it is diluted 400 times the distinct 'milk' crystal becomes stronger, even though there is less actual milk – if any – left in the water.

Quite apart from their ability to retain information, water molecules are stores of extraordinary energy. One litre of water is enough to keep a standard 60 watt bulb burning for about 100 hours.

A German engineer, Theodor Schwenk, talks of water as a receptive, almost separate, 'sense organ'. When a static body of water moves, even if you shake a bottle of it, it becomes more receptive. Schwenk, prepared several identical bottles of water and mechanically shook samples at 15-minute intervals before, during and after an eclipse. When the sun came out he popped wheat grains into the bottles and left them to germinate. The wheat in water shaken at the time of the eclipse grew far less than those in the water shaken before or after.

In 1996 at the Californian Institute of Technology, internationally respected theoretical physicist Shui-lin Lo PhD discovered an odd characteristic of water when he diluted a substance to the extreme. Lo found that odd ice crystals formed in the water when shaken. They had unusual electrical forces and did not 'melt' at room temperature. Verified by 2D electron microscope and atomic force 3D microscope these have been called I_E crystals, ice with an electrical field.

In trials with statistical odds against any difference at over 1,000 to 1, barley seeds have grown better in water held by healers.

Water is truly amazing, it breaks the rules of chemistry, physics and biology, and everything depends on it. It is the world's busiest substance, and it is ceaselessly moving within itself, without end.